101 Things to Do with a

Vibrator

101 THINGS
TO DO WITH A
VIBRATOR

MARISA BENNETT

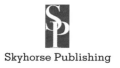

Skyhorse Publishing

Skyhorse Publishing books may be purchased in bulk at special discounts for sales promotion, corporate gifts, fund-raising, or educational purposes. Special editions can also be created to specifications. For details, contact the Special Sales Department, Skyhorse Publishing, 307 West 36th Street, 11th Floor, New York, NY 10018 or info@skyhorsepublishing.com.

Skyhorse® and Skyhorse Publishing® are registered trademarks of Skyhorse Publishing, Inc.®, a Delaware corporation.

Visit our website at www.skyhorsepublishing.com.

10 9 8 7 6 5 4 3 2 1

Library of Congress Cataloging-in-Publication Data is available on file.

Cover design by David Ter-Avanesyan
Cover art by CSA-Printstock/Getty Images

Paperback ISBN: 978-1-5107-6894-9
Hardcover ISBN: 978-1-62914-526-6
Ebook ISBN: 978-1-62914-840-3

Printed in China

table of contents

Introduction: Getting Buzzed

Electrify your sexual pleasure by exploring the world of vibrating sex toys! From small things that hum to complex toys that flick, rotate, swivel, and penetrate, find out everything you need to know to get your buzzworthy playtime charged up! Included are how-tos for a wide range of innovative sex toys, creative scenarios in which to use them, beautiful photography to showcase various toys, and even an erotica excerpt for inspiration! Whether you are a solo rider looking to intensify your Os and explore new sensations, or a part of a couple that wants to tease and please one another, *101 Things to Do with a Vibrator* will show you creative ways to entice, tempt, and vibe your way to incredible orgasms!

Wand Vibes: The Usual Suspects

The Care and Keeping of Vibrators

Choosing Your Material

Choosing your vibrator is so much more than just picking the prettiest one that you think will give you the most O power. They range in price and in texture, so it is important to know your options before you commit to a purchase. Vibrators are typically made from plastic, latex, cyberskin, jelly, and silicone. Below is a list of pros and cons for each:

PLASTIC: Plastic vibrators are super low priced and offer hard-as-a-rock penetration. They are safe with all types of lubricants and are super easy to clean. The not so sexy side of plastic vibrators is that while they might give you a good buzz, they are cheaper in quality and have shorter lifespans. The texture can be great for a quickie, but the hard material can be harsh on your lady parts and less intuitive with more complex areas like the g-spot and clitoris.

LATEX: Latex vibrators, like plastic vibrators, are great for the girl who wants it hard, but they also offer a softer texture so you don't feel like you're fucking a flashlight. They're slightly better quality and a tiny bit more expensive, but the flexibility will feel a little more natural. Latex vibrators are soft and a little porous, so you will need to use a water-based lube for each sexy session. Of course, if you are allergic to latex, using a latex vibrator is A BAD IDEA, so save yourself from a mortifying ER visit and choose another material!

JELLY: This is where vibrators get interesting! Jelly materials have given way for some unique and exotic vibrator designs to make your "you" time so much more fun. Jelly vibrators are mid-range in terms of price and easy to clean. They are pliable but firm, just the way a hard cock should be! There is some controversy over jelly vibrators containing phthalates, which is a substance in plastic that makes it more pliable. Phthalates have been found to cause health risks, ranging from minor irritation to severe health problems, so it is important to always look for the "phthalate-free" label when making a purchase.

CYBERSKIN: This high-end material gives the look and feel of real penetration. Cyberskin vibrators are generally firm in the way that latex toys are, but soft and smooth like the jelly material. These amazing vibrators will get you to your peak pleasure spot, but they require extra attention once you are finished and ready to clean them.

SILICONE: The gods of sex are smiling! Silicone vibrators are the premiere material for your buzzing pleasure. They are incredibly high quality, durable, hygienic, and will have a long lifespan if cared for properly. Silicone is certainly the top tier in vibrator quality, so they are priced accordingly. These kinds of vibrators will put a dent in your wallet in the short term, but are a good investment for your pleasure time in the long term.

Choosing the Right Lubricant

Using lubricants with your vibrator will bring your sexy session from satisfying to out of this world. The slippery sensation will get your engines revving much faster, but it will also allow you to continue riding your way to bliss a lot longer. There are some important things to note while choosing your lube, though! You would think that buying a lubricant would be a no-brainer, but the lubricant you buy can make all the difference in the lifespan of your sex toys, and can also determine how well your own body reacts to each hot rendezvous with your vibrator.

WATER-BASED: These lubricants are by far the best to buy because they are easy to clean (no oily residue), are safe for all vibrator materials, and do not create irritation on your skin.

OIL or PETROLEUM-BASED: Super fun! Unfortunately, these lubricants can corrode the sex toy material, particularly latex. Some people might experience irritation on their skin, as well.

SILICONE-BASED: Great for nearly every toy, this lubricant is sleek. They should never be used with a silicone sex toy though, because the material works against itself and can break down.

Cleaning and Storage

Cleaning your sexy toys is the most important factor in keeping yourself healthy and maintaining the quality of the toy itself. Because many vibrators are made from softer materials that are more porous, they are more prone to spreading bacteria and germs if they are not cleaned properly. Maintenance is super easy, and most toys just require a cleaning with a hot soapy towel. For anal play, sterilize your vibrator afterwards with rubbing alcohol or anti-bacterial soap to prevent cross-contamination, or use a condom.

Plastic toys can be wrapped in a clean towel and stored in a dry place, but more rubbery materials should be stored in a lint-free cloth like linen, silk, or a velvet bag. Remove batteries from your toys when you store them to maintain the best battery life.

PLASTIC: Soap and water or sex toy cleaner.

LATEX: Mild soap and water or sex toy cleaner.

JELLY: Mild soap and water or sex toy cleaner.

CYBERSKIN: Mild soap and water, Cyberskin cleaner, or sex toy cleaner. Dry with talcum power rather than rubbing with a towel to prevent breakdown of the material.

SILICONE: Soap and water or sex toy cleaner.

J

Wand Vibrators

A standard wand vibrator may not have all the bells and whistles, but it sure gets the job done. With a long, thick, hard shaft, a traditional vibrator fills you where you need to be filled and adds a euphoric buzz to pleasure what it cannot reach. The hum of a vibrator is constant and steady so that your sultry spots and clitoris get the steady attention they need. There are few limits to a traditional vibrator, so get naughty and kinky! Arch yourself over the end of your bed and slide the lubricated vibrator in from behind. Lie down on silk sheets and rub your pussy while you let the vibrator fill you. Lower yourself onto it and sit in a yoga pose, allowing the vibrations and the firm shaft to gradually take you over the edge. These vibrators have endless potential to take you to erotic heights!

2

Prolonged Pleasure for One

The tried and true use for a vibrator, this is the gold standard of self-sustained ecstasy. Whether you prefer a standard vibrator or like to get fancy with a heated clitoris tickler and rotating head, the best way to begin is by starting slowly and by making it last. Not all orgasms are created equal, so jumping into full power right away will be all sizzle and no steak. Start off by running the vibrator on a low setting everywhere but where you want it most. Run the vibrator along the inside of your legs and hips, and then settle it next to your outer lips so that the residual vibrations tease your clitoris. Turn the setting up slowly higher, moving from one side to the other, but delay hitting your clitoris. Bring the setting back down to a lower speed, and slowly ease it inside. By altering the settings each time you're close to orgasm, your pleasure will last longer and the orgasm will be more intense. Don't let the vibrator do all the work, slide it in and out at your preferred pace. Let it lean against your clitoris to get the full force of the vibrations, or go in deeply to hit your g-spot. Giving yourself these long-lasting sessions will feel amazing, but it will also get you comfortable with your body, making you feel sexy and confident in all of your sexual adventures.

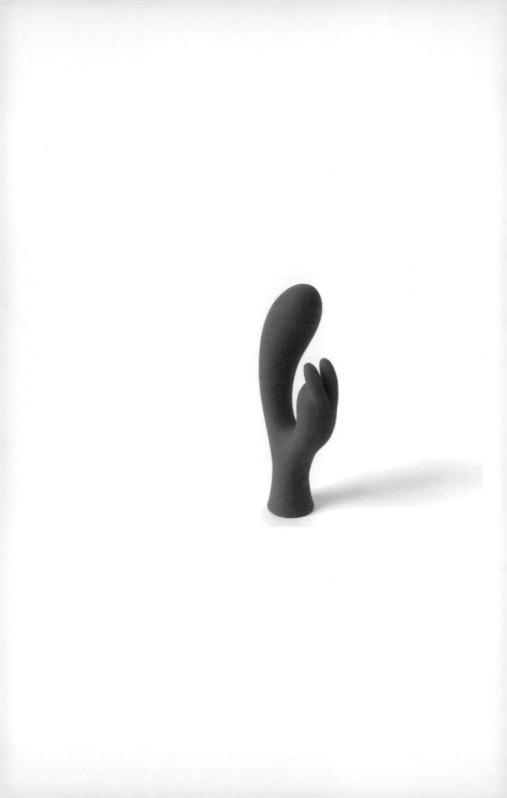

3

Thumper–The Rabbit Vibrators

Rabbit vibrators represent sexual innovation at its most complex, but more importantly, at its most orgasmic! This amazing tool has the smooth and hard feel of the real thing but has the technology to do what the real thing cannot! Most rabbit vibrators have a thick shaft that rotates in a cylindrical motion. This means that while you get the traditional, sensual fill of a vibrator, the mechanics rub circular pressure around the inside of your vagina. Many rabbit vibrators also have beads towards the base of the shaft, which add an extra element of sensual texture to fill you with ecstasy. The vibrator itself has "bunny ear" extensions that rhythmically pad against the clitoris for a mind-blowing, all-inclusive pathway to erotic bliss. This vibrator is so intense that you can just sit back and let it take you to orgasmic heights, or you can get creative and incorporate it into elaborate fantasies. Try leaning the humming bunny ears against the outer pussy lips to tease yourself, and slowly move to trail it along your clitoris. Get worked up and slide the full force of the vibrator into your pussy, allowing the g-spot massagers and bunny ears to work together and bring you an orgasm that makes your whole body shake!

𝔂

Just the Tip

One of the most amazing parts of a rabbit vibrator is the number of ways that it can pleasure you. Just because the rabbit is multitasking, though, does not mean that you have to do everything all at once. The best orgasms always come from a slow, intense build-up, and sometimes rabbits can take you over the edge too quickly for a superficial O. One way to prevent this is by limiting the elements in the rabbit vibrator, and bringing them all together closer to the end. Start off by lubricating the rabbit, even rubbing yourself with your wet fingers to get warmed up. Slide the tip of the rabbit into your warm pussy, and switch on the rotating head. The rotations will feel erotic and different and get you worked up to want the whole thing. Let's face it—sometimes the intensity is so amazing, that you just want to get fucked, and hard. So allowing a little time for teasing with *just the tip* will make when you finally take the whole girth into your hot pussy out of this world!

5

G-Spot Genius

While the clitoris may just be the greatest gift given to womankind, the g-spot is the difference between a great orgasm and a *fucking* great orgasm. For a deep, whole-body orgasm, g-spot vibrators focus on the deepest parts of a woman, with a rounded, rotating tip that is totally devoted to bringing you intense, sensual bliss. Slide your lubricated g-spot vibrator in deep, start off on a slow speed, and allow the rotations to massage the soft walls of your vagina. The intense rotations will work you into a sensual, slow trajectory toward a deep-feeling orgasm. To intensify these sensations, clench your kegel muscles so that your pleasure zone builds against the rotating head. The muscles will work together to build a full, internal orgasm that you will feel through your whole body!

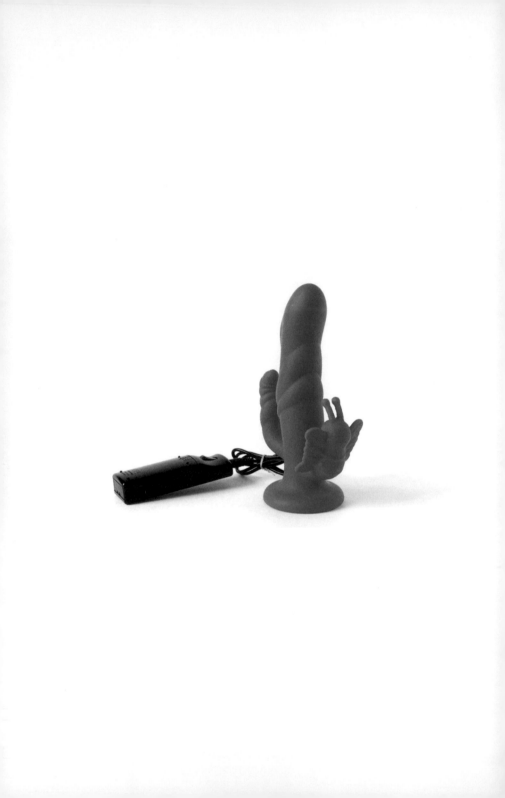

6

The Real Thing

Many vibrators have luxurious designs and soft contours to make you feel like you and your ecstasy are a part of a work of art. Other vibrators take the natural approach and provide the girth, coloring, and anatomically correct veins to get you hot. For the look and feel of a real cock (without the strings attached of a real cock!), fill yourself with an au naturel vibrator. Run your hands along the realistic shaft, enjoying the look and feel of the hard dick that lies before you! The best part of these vibrators is that you can make them do what you want, without any fear of it thrusting with the wrong rhythm or coming before you are ready! This cock makes sure *you* come first but is a sexy, realistic way to pleasure yourself.

7

The Real Thing—Three-Way

Threesomes can be fun, but they are also super complicated and have the power to destroy relationships. So have a threesome without having a threesome! Give your guy control and tell him to incorporate a natural-looking vibrator into your hot sex session. Tell him to trade off fucking you with his own shaft, as well as the natural-looking shaft that vibrates! Let him feel like he is in control by allowing him to pleasure you with the natural vibrator—watch it slide in and out of you as it sends humming vibrations throughout your pussy. Let it rest and slip him inside you to show him how hot you've gotten. Go back and forth between the two shafts to lengthen your rendezvous. Allowing him to use a toy on you will make him super hot, and you get the undivided attention of two hard men!

8

Sexy Photo Shoot

The Internet is an abyss of pornographic videos and sexy photos, but if imagery is what gets you going, it is always steamiest when the one in the frame is someone you are sleeping with. Whether looking at photos of your partner or yourself are what get you in the mood, a sexy vibrator photo shoot is hot and thrilling because it is just so naughty. Get into the lace, silk, or leather that makes you feel sexiest, or skip the lingerie altogether and go straight for the hardcore nudity. Since you will be incorporating your vibrator, you may want to choose automatic settings on your camera so that you (or your partner, if it is a couple's activity) do not have to keep making adjustments. Get deep into your hot mood by imagining that the camera is not even there, massage your body and let the vibrator in. Get up close and personal with the images, and let the lens capture your curves and sweet spots. Before you let yourself climax, look through the photos and turn yourself on with the simultaneous visual and vibrating pleasure. Photos are an amazing way to get into the mood and satisfy you from beginning to blissful end.

Photo and Internet Safety

Yes, photos are fucking sexy! It turns anyone on to take them and to look at them, whether you are solo or with a partner, but there are very real risks to getting it on with a lens in the room. No matter how much you trust your partner or yourself, accidents can happen, flash drives can get lost, cameras can get stolen, and, even more sadly, partners can take images and upload them to "revenge porn" websites in a moment of anger. Having photos of yourself in an intimate scenario is completely normal, but those images are **forever** and can affect your daily life, your career, and your relationships if they are put in the wrong hands. This does not mean you can't have a little fun, it just means you should **take precautions:**

• When taking photos that you know are being "saved for later," make sure your face or major identifying characteristics are not shown in the photography.

• If you have full videos or images of your face, never trust that they are going to get deleted just because you asked nicely: watch them get deleted and cleared from the computer's trash can or the camera's memory card.

• Never save intimate photos or videos on the Internet. While many photo websites have security measures and are password protected, computer whizzes and internet hackers are very good at what they do and can hack into these sites, steal your sexy photos, and do with them what they please.

9

One for Me, One for You

If you are experimenting with vibrators with a partner, have a little fun with it! Both of you should choose a vibrator that really entices you. Work the vibrators in to your lusty liaison, but don't rush! Just when you really start to build up some serious passion, trade places. Let your partner use the vibrator you chose on you, and then stop and start pleasuring your partner with the toy they chose. Switch off repeatedly, delaying orgasm for both of you so that your arousal becomes overwhelming! When you have pleasured each other for so long that it becomes just too much, get each other off simultaneously with the chosen toys. The build-up will allow for an amazing release of pleasure that satisfies both of you.

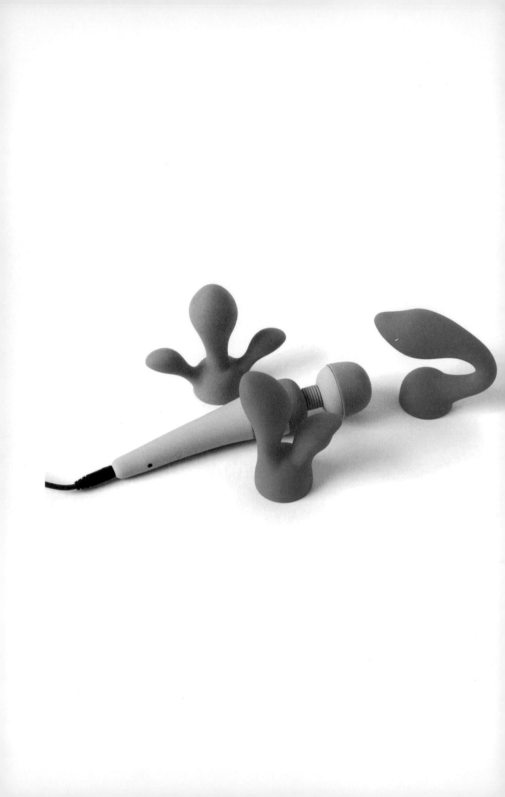

10

Getting Attached

A single vibrator does not mean a single sensation. Some vibrators come with multiple attachments that allow you to replace the head of the vibrator depending on your mood. Varying in shapes and size, from large orbs, to swan-like heads, to triple-action heads, each provides a unique way to engage in your hot session. The most complex attachments, like those with three prongs, are for the lover of multitasking! The massagers allow for clitoral, vaginal, and anal stimulation all at the same time so that you can never get bored! Get exploratory with each vibrator head and make a game of it. Choose the head you like best and let it give you its undivided attention, or switch through each of the heads during a single lust session to give yourself ever-changing bliss!

11

Race to the Finish

Records are made to be broken, so it's time to get competitive about your orgasmic endurance. Choose your favorite sex toy and get to work on getting the high score for hitting your passionate peak. Most women hit the edge fastest from pleasuring their clitoris, so give it your undivided attention. Rub your fingers in circles over your clitoris and insert your vibrator deep inside, putting it on its highest setting. Switch places and place the heavy vibrations over your clit, and slide your fingers into your pussy. Make the switch often or stick with what gets you hottest. Work up a sweat! Get into giving your pleasure hub attention from every angle, and bring yourself over the edge. After your first O, keep going! The first one is always the most work, so count your way to your peak as many times as you can before you are totally exhausted. Sometimes a girl just needs rapid-fire orgasms!

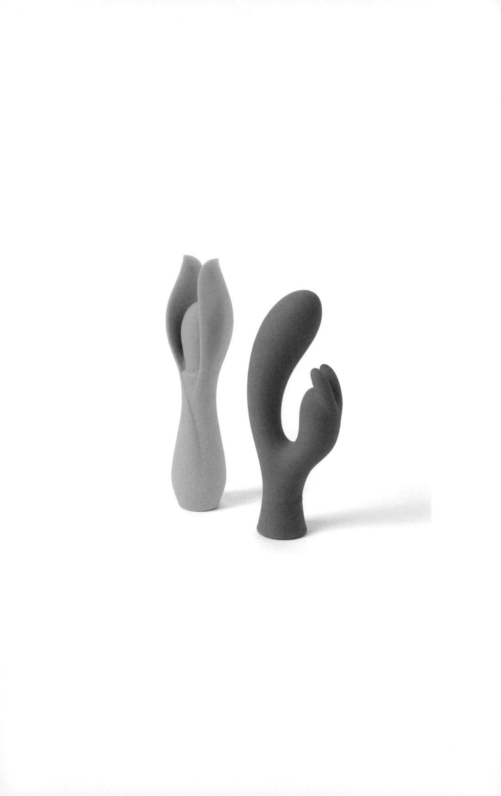

12

Edward Buzzer Hands

Get tied to your vibrators! With a partner or solo, choose two completely different kinds of vibrators and fasten them to your hands using strong tape or rope. If you are solo, just make sure to not tie them too tightly so that you can get free later. You are letting the vibrators become an extension of your hands for optimal pleasure! If you are with a partner, the goal is that you are not allowed to remove the vibrators until you have given them a certain number of orgasms. You set the number, but it has to be more than one! This fun way to approach a vibing puts a little humor into your love session but also ensures that everyone leaves happy and satisfied again and again!

13

Literary Love

Erotic literature is nothing new, but recent bombshell books have led to a sexual awakening amongst readers who had never before crossed over to the romance and erotica aisles. Go on a sexy reading adventure and select a wide range of novels and short stories to pique your fancy and broaden your sexual horizons. From paranormal romance about shape-shifting lovers, to futuristic love stories on a moon commune, to firefighters, gay cowboys, erotic twists to fairy tales, or regency ladies of pleasure, there are no limits to exploring the pages of a hot erotica story! Try a different short story every night or let your fantasies get wrapped up over the course of a whole novel, enhancing your sexual pleasure. Delve into the storylines and imagine yourself as the damsel or the dominatrix. Oh, and bring your vibrator!

14

Get Shakespearean

Erotic stories and tales of intense sexual rendezvous needn't be left to all the former English majors. Get creative and write your own story of erotic thrillers and sensual utopias! The act of writing inspires the imagination and lets you explore your most intimate desires, so let it all flow onto the page. The further you get into your lusty literature, the more intense the satisfaction will be when you incorporate your pleasure vibes into the storyline! Pleasure yourself while you come up with ideas, or let your passion build until the end and hit your climax when your characters do! Read your stories back to yourself or share them with a partner and bring your sexual creativity to life.

15

Pride and Prejudice and Orgies

Sexy fan fiction! If you don't have a creative bone in your body, but you *want* a bone in your body, try piggybacking onto your favorite non-sexual stories and adding a little smut! You do not need to be a writer to add a little fuckery to a plot, so start small. Take a copy of a book or adjust a PDF, adding your own endings, naughty phrases, and sexual romps to the text. If you want to get a little more creative, read through your favorite novel and come up with your own twist to the storyline using the same characters and setting. Remember, this is for your personal pleasure, so do not post or publish a story online that has been taken from another author. The point is to have fun and add a little excitement to your vibe lifestyle! Read the stories over and over and get yourself hot for the next time you want the hum of a sex toy against your hot spots!

16

Cinéma Érotique

It isn't a far leap from vibrator play to watching a dirty film.
Instead of choosing your typical porno, try broadening your
horizons by watching a foreign porno while you vibe. Whether
you have a particular longing for a Parisian, or think a Latin
lover sounds enticing, listening to the erotic sounds of another
language is like listening to a sensual rhythm. While you may
not understand the words, the sexuality and cadence of the
actors' voices will heighten your senses and lure you into the
storyline. Let a different kind of naughty film excite you and take
you to places you have never been!

17

Love Rider

Reaching your sexual summit with a vibrator can oftentimes be a passive experience. You lay back and let the vibes take you where you want to go, but sometimes, rather than *getting* fucked, it is so much hotter to be the one doing the fucking. For these times, try a vibrator with a suction cup base. Place it on a clean, firm surface, and consider putting soft pillows under your knees. If you chose a multi-function vibrator, work your way to ecstasy as you let the clitoral stimulator perk you up, or tease your ass with the back-end stimulator while you fuck the shaft. This satisfying toy lets you be in charge while you ride your way to sexy peaks!

18

Spin the Vibrator

Spin the bottle is a timeless classic, but it lacks the kind of spice that leads to wild sex play and pulsing orgasms. So trade out this old-timey game and add some kink! On an oversized piece of paper, draw a large clock. Instead of numbers, line the clock with kinky tasks to do with your vibe toys. From oral, to 69ing, to paddles, and feather ticklers, each of these tasks should supplement your favorite vibrating toy. Use a vibrating bullet to magnify cunnilingus or head, or use a vibrator with a rotating head while you get smacked with a riding crop! The options are endless, but the anticipation of what you will get next will be thrilling and hot!

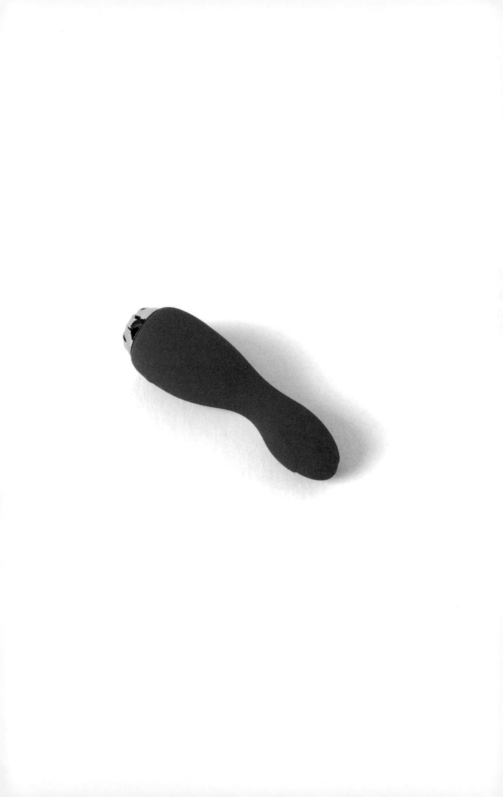

19

Twist and Shout

This game is Twister, but naked, sexy, and electrified! Play a round (or several) of classic Twister, but set erotic regulations. Insert a bullet or a small vibrator while you bend and twist, and see how long you can go before your knees give out from pleasure. Get tangled with your partner and slide against each other's naked bodies to get worked up and feeling sexy. Get wrapped around and exposed in vulnerable angles and use a finger vibrator or a lubricated standard vibe to entice, distract, and get yourself or your partner off. This version of this fun game is ultra hot and will undoubtedly lead to desire levels that are not just passionate, but incredibly fun!

20

Sexual Growth

Break out your erotic arsenal for this hot step-by-step climb to the climax! Arrange your toys from smallest to largest. Start with ben wa balls, and slide them into your pussy. Tighten your kegel muscles around the hard orbs and feel your inner warmth pulse and intensify. Remove the balls and insert a small bullet or egg vibrator. Move your pelvis in circles so that the humming egg massages deep inside at all angles. Remove the egg and slide in a small shaft vibrator. Slip it in and out and feel it slide and vibe against the inside of your vagina. Make the switch to a g-spot vibrator, allowing the rotating head to reach your deepest parts and enhance your bliss. Make the move to a rabbit vibrator, letting it take you to the peak as it penetrates you hard and erotically from the inside and hums against your clitoris on the outside. If you love size, move on to an extra large vibrator to fill you completely and experience the tightness of your pussy around the shaft as you hit your sexual peak!

21

Slip into Something Less Comfortable

The fashion industry has made it seem like sexy outfits, lingerie, and dominatrix leather are meant for the pleasure of everyone else but the person wearing them. So not true! One of the greatest parts of getting dressed so that you can get *undressed*, is the confidence it gives you in your body and how sexy you feel. Pick out something super hot or super kinky that you might not wear for someone else. Slip into racy Catwoman leather and swish a riding crop. Wear crotch-less panties and nipple tassels to make you feel wickedly wanton. Accent your curves with hot red lace. Dress up as the naughty forensic scientist who needs to explore some anatomy. Whatever entices you, you should approach this scenario by thinking about what makes you feel sexy, and not what you think makes other people hot. If you feel sexy, you will turn yourself on and feel amazing. Get into the mood of your outfit choice and let your vibrator fulfill every desire!

22

Flipping the Switch

Get your favorite vibrator ready by rubbing it down with a sensual lubricant and begin to massage yourself manually. Without turning the vibrator on, slide it up and down on the outside of your vagina—along your outer and inner pussy lips and sliding against your clitoris. Slip the vibrator inside your pussy—still without turning it on. Get worked up simply from the slick sensation of the hard shaft in and against you. Thrust hard and fast and put all of your effort into feeling the force of the shaft. When you feel like you are on the edge of your climax, turn the vibrations on full force to send you careening over the blissful summit!

23

Internette Roulette

Sometimes even *choosing* a toy to get you off is an overwhelming task. Do you buy a bullet vibrator for an intimate buzz or a multi-functioning rabbit vibrator with a beaded shaft? Is a vibrator with a curved head better than a vibrator with a bulbous one? Will a clitoris tickler make everything better, or will it take away from how hot it feels to be penetrated with a hard shaft? For big questions like these, you should take big risks! While searching for sex toys on the web, go to a page with a wide selection. Move the page up and down quickly so that it is difficult to distinguish between toys. Close your eyes, wiggle the mouse or cursor, and whichever toy you land on will be the one you purchase. (If you land on something you already own, try again.) This maneuver will force you to experiment with toys you may not have taken a second notice of earlier and feel new sensations that will surprise and amaze you!

Small Vibes: Little Toys with a Big Buzz

Introduction: Starting Small

Vibrators come in an almost endless number of shapes and sizes, which means, whatever your pleasure, you'll likely be able to find a vibrator that fits you just right. If you're feeling intimidated by some of the big gyrating devices you see on the front page of the sex toys website, you might want to start with something small. Luckily there are plenty of little wonders that will blow your mind!

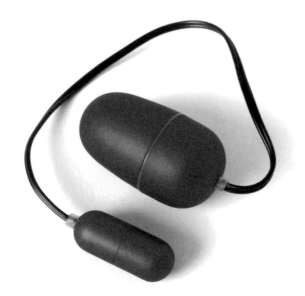

23

Egg and Bullet Vibes

While the wand vibrator usually gets top billing as the "classic" sex toy shape, egg or bullet vibes give them a run for their money in versatility. These small toys can pack a punch, and you can use them on just about any erogenous zone you'd like! As the name suggests, these vibes are small, usually between two and three inches in length and less than an inch in diameter, and they come in a variety of oblong shapes. Many bullet vibes are controlled by a switch that is attached to the vibrator with wires, which allows you to change the setting without moving the vibrator and gives you some interesting options for couple's play! Other models work wirelessly, with the batteries and on/off switch in the vibe itself. Some fancier models even let you control the vibrations with a wireless switch! Which model is best for you depends a lot on what you plan to do with it. These things are seriously multi-use, so be creative!

25

Who Holds the Remote?

Here's a fun way to start off your night—trade the TV remote for the one on your bullet vibrator! The rule is you take turns with your partner: one of you holds the remote to control the speed and intensity of the vibe, and the other holds the toy in place. Switch off whenever you switch positions! This works best if your toy has multiple settings so you can really change it up. Incorporate this tip whenever you play with your toy: it gives you the chance to play with your partner, and show each other just where you like it. This keeps both partners involved and engaged, even when the action is focused on just one of you. Make a house rule that whoever holds the remote turns up the intensity based on how turned on they are, so as you drive your partner crazy they can return the favor.

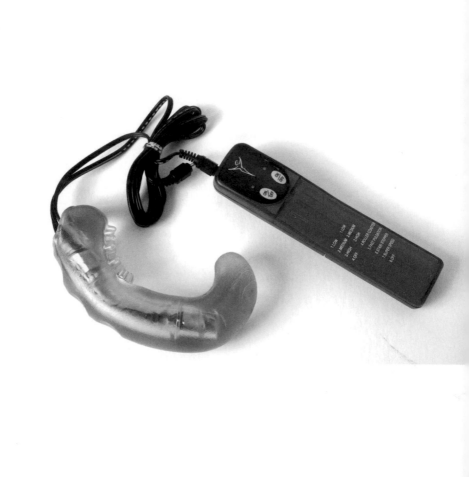

26

Battery-Powered Pregame

Vibrations feel good all over, so why relegate your vibe to only the obvious places? Incorporate your little vibrators into your foreplay routine. Use the vibe on your partner as you touch, stroke, and caress each other to get revved up. If your toy is small enough, you can palm it and use it to supercharge your strokes. Roll your vibe over your skin, paying special attention to your favorite sensitive spots, like nipples or inner thighs. Alternate the strength and speed of the vibration depending on what feels best: a stronger buzz will work great on areas with thicker skin, like on your ass or thighs, while a lighter touch will do the trick for thin-skinned places like your nipples. Hand the vibe to your partner to let him take you for a ride, or put on a show and teach him how you like it!

27

Jacked Up

Vibrators are for pussies, right? Not so: some penises also can benefit from the buzz! Next time he's jacking it, he can jack it up by adding a little vibration, either solo or with an extra hand. Start with the vibrator set on low speed, and experiment with different sensations all around his penis. Try palming the vibe or holding the cord between your fingers so you can give him a buzz while you stroke him. If your vibe is nice and cylindrical, try rolling it gently against his shaft, moving from his balls all the way to the head of his penis. Check in with your partner as you go to see what he likes best! Once your explorations have him moaning, you can make him yours with this hot finishing move: grab his dick with one hand, while you hold the vibrating bullet in your other. As you stroke him off, drag the vibe down along the base of his penis, using it to stimulate his penis, balls, and anywhere else he wants as you finish off his favorite kind of high five.

28

Buzzworthy Oral

Electrify your oral technique with a little vibe. As you start to go down on your partner, run the vibrator along all of his erogenous zones. Play lightly along his nipples, down his chest, and along the inside of his hips. Take him in your mouth, and bring the vibrator—whether a standard issue or a small egg— and rest it against your cheek as you perform your sultry oral. The light vibrations to go with your tongue and lips will expose him to a whole new side of oral bliss. If you want to get even naughtier, try one of two things: While you go down on him, start using the vibrator on yourself. Let him know how good you're both feeling, and even let him in on the action. If you like it best when you're in total control, take the vibrator to new places. As you tongue him down, bring the vibrator lightly against his scrotum. Let it linger, and then bring it back to his perineum. The vibrating sensations in this [nearly] naughtiest of locations will have him going wild.

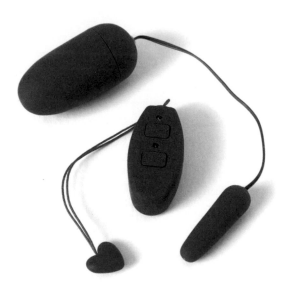

29

Back Door Buzzer

The bullet vibe is a great toy for adding some back door buzz to your fun! We all have plenty of sensitive nerve endings in our butts, and you don't need penetration to play. When you're getting down and dirty, slide the egg vibe between your cheeks and rest it right on your asshole. Rev up the vibrations and you're in for a ride! For best results, combine with other fun stimulation, with your hands, with another toy, or with a friend! Try this during foreplay or while you are going down on your partner. Have your partner start by using the little vibe to gently massage your butt cheeks. As you start to relax, have your partner slowly make his way to your asshole, keeping the vibrations low. Have him keep drawing circles around your asshole as your play, and as you get into it, don't be afraid to lean into the toy so the buzz hits the right spot! Once your partner finishes you off, it's time to switch places and try it again!

30

Two to Tango

I always say it takes two to tango, and a little toy can help keep you both grooving while you're orally pleasing your mate. Watching you writhe with pleasure will drive your partner crazy—and keep you occupied, too! Have your partner control the remote while you hold the vibe in place, and then use your other hand and your mouth to stimulate him. You can try it semi-69 style, and arrange your body so he can hold the vibe and play with you while you give him a blowjob. It's hotter doing it together—who likes to wait their turn?

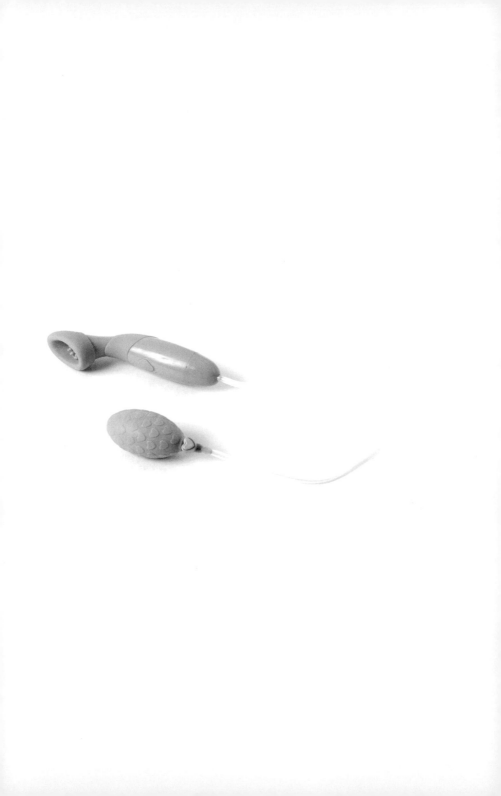

31

Inner Peace

People tend to think little vibes like the egg or bullet vibrator are for external pleasure only, but like I said, these little vibrators are seriously versatile, and you can create some amazing sensations if you think outside (or, rather, inside?) the box! Just lube up your bullet and slide it into your vagina—don't forget to turn it on first, unless it has a remote! The smaller vibrator works great for internal stimulation, and unlike other larger vibes, you are free to move into different positions without worrying about your vibrator falling out or getting in the way! While your toy is buzzing away, you or your partner can stimulate your clitoris, delivering a double dose of pleasure!

32

Triple-A Oral

Supercharge your orgasm by combining two of a girl's favorite things: vibration and oral! Start by using the vibe for foreplay: take turns with your partner holding the vibe, and work your way from your clitoris to your vagina. When you are warmed up, help your partner to slowly slide the little vibe into your vagina. You can use a little lube if you'd like, but your partner may prefer you choose something flavored. While your partner goes down on you, grab your remote control, and adjust the speed and intensity as he moves around. While his mouth is busy, he can use his hands to play with the bullet vibe: have him gently push the toy toward the front wall of your vagina to stimulate your g-spot, or tug on the wire or string to move the vibe back and forth. You might find it feels best just to leave the toy where it is, and let him concentrate on his oral technique!

33

Stringing Along

Try this fun technique for manual play with the bullet vibe, either solo or with your partner. The trick is to move your vibe using only the attached wire or strap, instead of holding the toy in your hand. This gives you less control over the buzzing vibe, making the sensations more unexpected and stimulating! Start with the vibrator on low, and rest the bullet right outside your vagina. Hold the cord a few inches from the bullet, and tug gently, so that the bullet bobs slightly against you. Drag the toy up toward your clitoris, then drag it up and over, and bring it back down to rest below your clit. Try to find a rhythm and keep it up for a bit, and turn the vibrator intensity up as you get more turned on. Let the cord go slack and have gravity roll the bullet down: try this in a few different positions to get the full effect! Change it up by lifting the bullet up and dangling it by the cord. Move the vibe up and down, tapping and buzzing specific parts of your pussy. If you are playing with your partner, take turns holding the remote and changing the speed: your partner can help supercharge your fun by turning up the intensity as you graze your most sensitive spots!

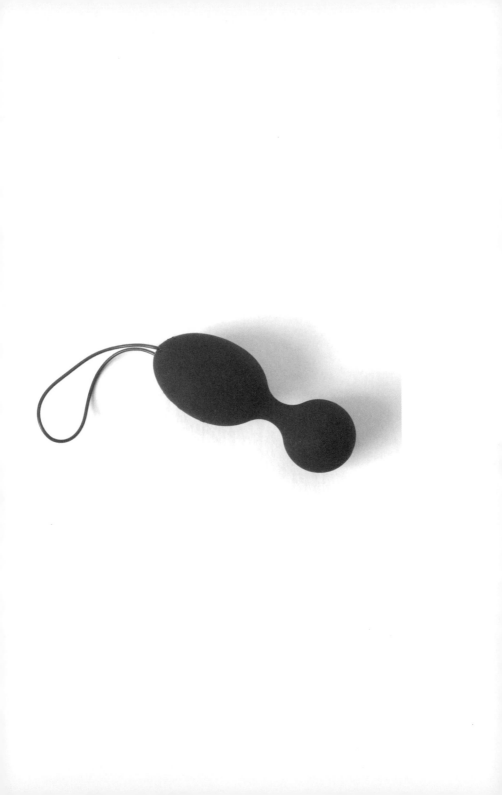

34

Buzz to Music

Grooving while you're getting down can be fun solo or with a partner! Just pick a track and turn up the volume. Use your hand to hold your bullet vibe in place and use the remote to choreograph your sensations. For fast-paced songs with a heavy beat, pulse your vibe in time to the bass. Resist the urge to speed up as you get yourself turned on! For a slower groove, use a sublet touch: instead of pulsing off and on, spin the controls to adjust the intensity as the music swells. Make the toy rumble on low to match the notes, then crank it on up when they're belting out the high notes. It'll be over long before the fat lady sings . . .

35

Eggcellent Rubdown

Bullet vibes are great for targeted fun, but for a solo sesh with a wider appeal, you may want to try a vibe a bit more on the "egg" side, as opposed to the smaller bullet models. A slightly bigger toy gives you less pinpoint precision, and more all-over vibration, which is just what you need for a leisurely romp with your favorite date, yourself! But don't just dive in; give yourself a nice long rubdown. Start by rolling the egg over your legs, moving toward the inside of your thighs. Move your way closer to your clitoris, and roll the egg in circles around your vulva. When you move in on your clitoris, use the oblong shape of the vibe to move the toy in interesting ways: roll it over your clit, and move it in more little circles to concentrate the buzz right where you want it.

36

Bullet in the Butt

Bullet vibes have so many different uses, and they are a fantastic way to add new sensations to your sexcapades! Many toy enthusiasts also use bullet vibe for anal play, and there are some bullet vibes made specifically for this purpose! It's always best to only put toys meant for anal play in your back door, but if you want to try your little bullet out, you will be better off if you only use bullets with a cord or strap to pull it out, and if you put the vibe in a condom, it helps for quick and easy clean up and toy retrieval at the end of your tryst! Check out page 140 for more butt play safety tips. If you are trying this on "her," try combining it with some mind-blowing oral: the intense stimulation of oral combined with a soft buzzing in the butt can result in some really fantastic orgasms! You can also try vaginal sex while she has the vibe in her butt: this is a great low-pressure way to try out some double-penetration action! A girl-on-top position will probably be most comfortable, or even doggy style, if he wants a good view of her backside.

And don't leave him out: some men say that an inserted bullet vibe is just the thing to hit your prostate—and it pairs quite well with a blow job, or some good old fashioned P-in-the-V sex. Doggy style is good here, too, or a slow and sensual missionary.

37

Double Bullet

Some bullet vibes come with multiple bullets attached to the remote, so you can have more buzz for your buck! These double-bullet vibes work just like the single-bullet version, but you can use them on multiple pleasure points at once, and control them all by the same remote! There is an almost endless number of ways for you to make this work for you. Stimulate her nipples and her clitoris at once (great for a speedy masturbation sesh or a special treat for you). Slide one inside your vagina, and use the other on your clitoris. Rub one against his erection while you use the other on your clitoris.

38

Two for One

Bullet vibes are great for solo use, and double bullet models are twice as nice! There are a ton of combinations you can try with this toy. Start by resting one bullet on your vagina (you'll want to try this while in a reclining position). Hold the other in your other hand, and use it to stimulate your clitoris. Alternate by moving one bullet up to your nipples, then trail it back down. You can slide one of the bullets inside of you, and let the other one roam. Don't forget to turn up the intensity on the remote!

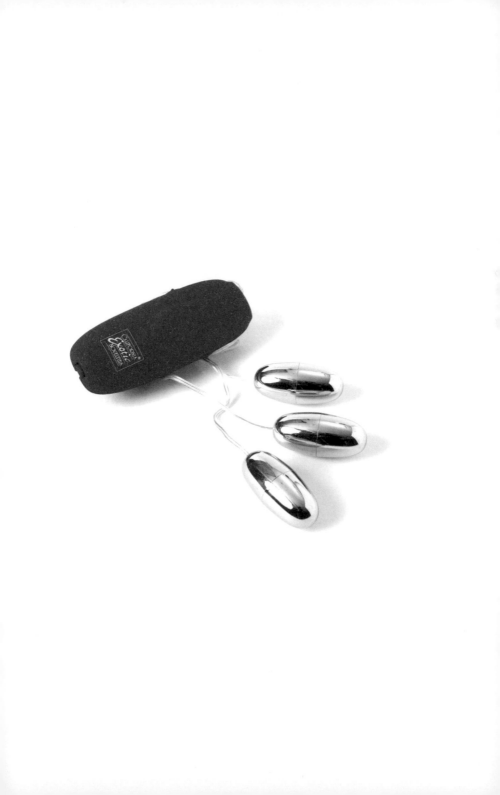

39

Three for Two

The sky's the limit for multiple bullet vibes—actually, three is pretty much the limit, and you typically won't find one of these with more than three bullets per remote. But you can have a lot of fun with three! There are plenty of configurations for you to try, and with three vibes, there's more than enough buzz to go around. Try inserting one vibe in your vagina, and then you and your partner hold the remaining two vibes. You can use them on each other, or put on a show! Or, use two bullets to play with him while he pleases you with the other one. You can use one bullet to stimulate his testicles while you stroke up and down his shaft with the other one. If your vibrator's cords are long enough, let the toys roam, and use one on his shaft while the other two stimulate your clitoris and nipples!

40

Ben Wa Buzz

Ben Wa balls have gained a bit of celebrity after being featured in the scorching BDSM erotica *50 Shades of Grey*. This little toy consists of two balls made of plastic or metal, each with a bit of weight to them. Not only are Ben Wa balls fun, they also act like little exercise weights for your kegel muscles, making you feel "tighter" for your partner, and giving you easier, more intense orgasms! Many women like Ben Wa balls because they give you a different sensation from a lot of sex toys: they fill you up and can stimulate your g-spot easily, creating the perfect counterpoint to clitoral stimulation. With vibrating Ben Wa balls, you kick your fun up to the next level! Just like with the bullet vibe, you lube these babies up and slide them in. You don't need any help to rock out with this toy. One good way to get going is to sit up with your legs closed and rock back and forth: this moves the balls around and helps to stimulate the sensitive nerves of your g-spot on the front wall of your vagina.

41

But Wait, There's More

Vibrating Ben Wa balls are fun for foreplay and other sexy games, but not as useful if you and your partner want to party together. Luckily, you can totally play with Ben Wa balls with a friend! Once the balls are in place and you're all warmed up, have him slowly enter you right along with the ben wa balls. Vaginas are plenty stretchy, and you'll have room for your toy and your man's monster cock (is he reading over your shoulder? That was for his benefit) if you move slowly. But if you're uncomfortable, you can also just insert one of the balls, and as long as you go slow, you'll be golden. Sex with Ben Wa balls is a treat for both partners: as he thrusts, the ball rolls against his shaft while it rubs you the right way, too!

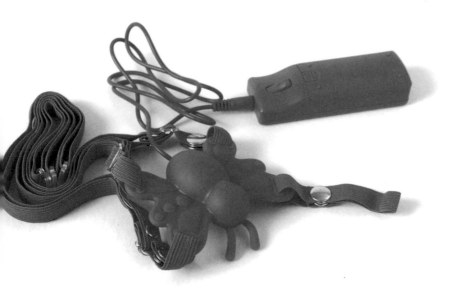

42

Butterfly Buzz

Bullet vibes and other small toys are super useful, but sometimes you want something hands-free, so that your hands can get busy doing something more fun than keeping a vibrator in place! If you want a toy that stays right where you want it, either for partner play or a solo sesh, try out a butterfly vibrator. These come in different makes and models, and are usually held in place with a harness, although some models also include suction, which helps keep the toy in place, and create even more stimulation by increasing blood flow. These toys also have a handy remote, either wireless or with a nice long cord that will let you lay back and enjoy while you adjust the settings.

43

Butterfly Bebop

There are very few vibes that are truly "hands free," which is what makes butterfly vibrators extra special and really easy to combine with other sexy fun! You can start with oral: with the vibe taking care of your clitoris, he'll be able to explore where else you like to be stroked. You can finish it there, or if you want penetration, you can jump into your favorite position: the vibe will stay put and give you an electric thrill while he pounds you! You can even combine this with other toys for a really wild experience! Use a dildo or another vibrator to fill you up and stroke your g-spot while the butterfly keeps your clit happy. Or try it with a vibrating butt plug for a buzz from both sides!

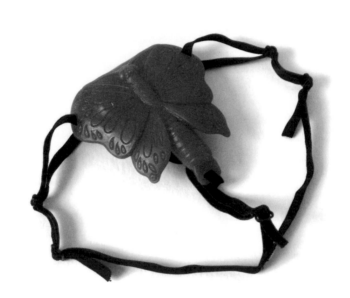

33

Hold My Hand

A ring vibe can help supercharge your touch, so give yourself a hand! You can play with your partner or on your own, because this toy works by sending the vibes through your fingers: you can work your moves the way you usually do, but with an extra jolt! Walk your fingers north and play with your nipples, then trace them down below the belt. The indirect buzz combined with your skilled and familiar fingers make for a unique new sensation. Or if you're playing with a partner, wrap your hands around his penis for a heavy-duty hand job, and take time to reach down to stroke his balls!

45

Mini Pick-Me-Up

Small vibes can pack a punch, so much so that you'll want to take yours with you! You can find many mini-massager vibes to fit your style and to fit in your purse. These little babies are made for discrete fun on the go, so take yours with you when you're on the move. Then, next time you need a pick-me-up, boost your day by getting down with your handy little toy! You can pop it in your pocket and take a morning walk, or sneak a few seconds alone in the office storage closet. Hey, it's healthier than taking a cigarette break, right?

Couple's Play

Introduction

Vibrations can be fun on their own, or you can bring some toys to bed and help supercharge your favorite positions! Some toys are best with a partner, too, and it's hard to play sex games alone. So grab your partner and get to bed for some hot vibrating fun!

46

Position: Doggy with Style

This position is easy to work with almost any vibrator, from big wand models to small bullet vibes. Start by using the toy to get you both warmed up: take turns using the vibe on each other and adjusting the speed and intensity. Once you're both turned on, position yourselves into the classic doggy pose. You'll need a free hand to wield your toy, so tuck a pillow under your upper body to help prop you up as he takes you from behind. It may be difficult to stay upright if you try to hold the toy yourself while in a hands-and-knees position, so let him give you a hand! Prop yourself up on both hands (or elbows, if you like that angle better), and let him hold the vibe. He can hold on to your hip with one hand while he brings his other hand around to your front to give you an electric reach-around. Once you've hit a good rhythm, you can reach back and help him find just the right spot!

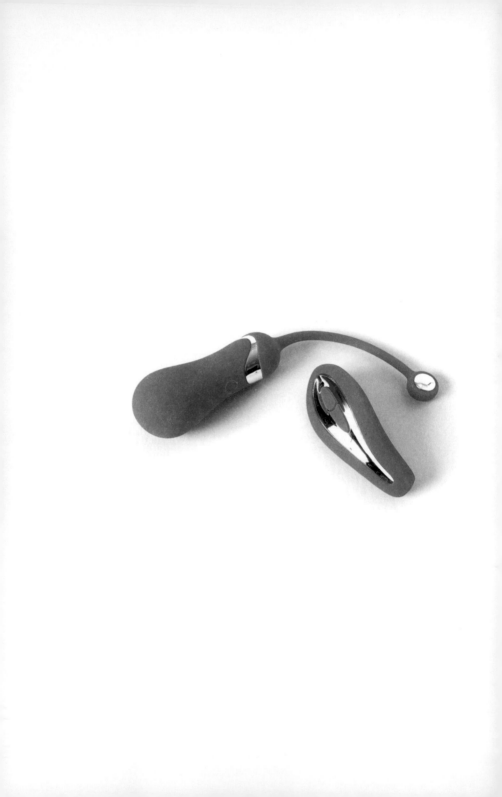

47

Position: Bend Over Buzzing

This rear-approach position is a modified doggy style, but this time you hold the vibe while he concentrates on the fucking. Position yourself so that you are on your knees with your upper body resting on the bed and your ass in the air. Use pillows under your hips and chest to get the right angle. He should be kneeling behind you and holding on to your hips to keep you both steady. Once you have a steady rhythm going, reach around and bring the vibe to your clitoris for a one-two punch! This is also a good angle for trying anal play or incorporating a butt plug.

48

Position: Ride 'Em Cowgirl

This position gives both partners a front-row seat to your own sexy rodeo! Use your favorite vibe to stimulate your clitoris while taking him for a ride. After you've both warmed up with some steamy foreplay, have your partner lie back on the bed and hop on in the Cowgirl position. As you start to move together, pull out your trusty toy and aim it right at your clitoris. Hold the vibe however is most comfortable for you and your position: with a smaller bullet vibe you can palm the toy and hold it against you for a less direct buzz, or you can cup it against you for more random buzzing. If you want a more targeted approach, try a wand vibe with a larger head: it will have more buzzy surface area so it won't matter as much if the toy gets jostled as you play. Depending on the type and strength of toy you're using, your man will get to enjoy the vibrations, too!

49

Position: Cowbuzz

Girl on top is always a winning move, and if you turn it around to reverse cowgirl, he gets to enjoy the buzz, too (and a nice view of your ass)! Start by getting comfortable and getting into position. Once you start to grind into him, pull out your favorite vibe. With an egg or bullet vibe, take turns stimulating your clitoris, his balls, and the base of his shaft as you move with him. Make sure to spend just enough time on each spot so you drive him wild before moving on to tickle the next sensitive spot. With a wand vibe, you have more space to play, so try to stimulate him and you at the same time. Hold the wand vibe so that you rub against it as you ride him and the tip of the vibe gently buzzes against his package.

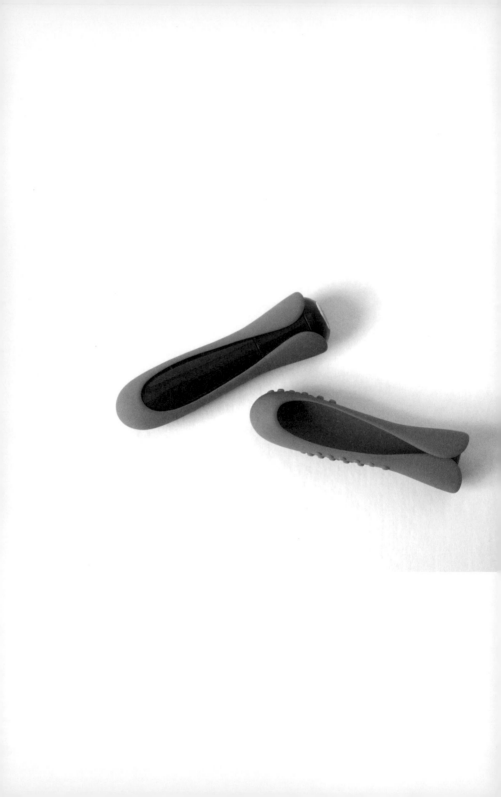

50

Position: Meeting in the Middle

Face to face positions are fun when you're using a toy, since part of the thrill of vibrators is watching them do their thing. So try this hot move that has you both within arm's reach of the action. Lay on your back with one knee up, and your other leg out in front of you. Have him kneel and straddle your straightened leg, and slide inside you. He can pull your bent leg closer to his chest to pull you closer to him and get good leverage. Now, just add vibes! You can use a wand vibe on your clitoris, with either of you holding the toy. Since you're so close, you could also use a bullet or egg vibe to play.

51

Position: Something's Between Us

This intimate position is just begging for a little vibe to make it even better. First, have him sit with his legs out in front of him. Climb on and sit on his lap, face to face with him. Wrap your legs around his torso as he slides into you. Now that you're both so neatly entwined, pull out a toy and rest or hold it right between you, near your clitoris. This position is good for deep, grinding sensations, so use the toy to add another level of sensation to your movement. Take turns positioning your vibe where it feels good: you can even take a break to tease your partner with the toy or trace it along his upper body.

52

Position: Tabled

This position is fun and naughty, and with toys added it can feel like a diabolically dirty science experiment! Find a piece of furniture that is about hip height for your man, like a bed or a table. Climb up and lay down with your hips right at the edge and have him enter you as you wrap your legs around his hips. Now you're ready for a very satisfying romp, and your man is perfectly positioned to reach all of your sensitive spots, and you are free to reach down and stimulate your clit, either with your hands or a handy vibe. For extra fun, have a few toys laid out on the table for effect. He can also step away from the table and walk around to touch you from above, play with the vibes, and maybe use them on your pussy or ass. Just add some soft restraints, and you are in for a wild time! Just don't forget to wash the table when you're done.

53

Position: Stairway Ride

Remember when you were a kid and you used to scoot down the stairs on your butt? This is just like that, but more fun. Find a private set of stairs (preferably in your home, but you do what feels right) and have him sit down. Sit on his lap, facing away from him and straddling one of his legs, while he enters you. Make sure you have your favorite vibe with you, and take turns using it to stimulate your clitoris. You can use the railing for extra leverage to help you move up and down. From this angle, you can push up against him to help him hit the right spot as you wield your toy.

54

Position: Electric Lap Dance

This position is super intimate, and puts you in the thrusting drivers seat. It's a bit of a tight fit, so you'll want to use a small toy, preferably one that stays in place on its own, like a hands-free butterfly vibe or a cock ring. Get your toy going, and then have your man sit in a sturdy chair. Straddle him and sit facing him, and slide him inside of you. Now you can use your feet to brace against the floor to move you against him. The closer you grind, the more you'll feel the buzzy toy between you!

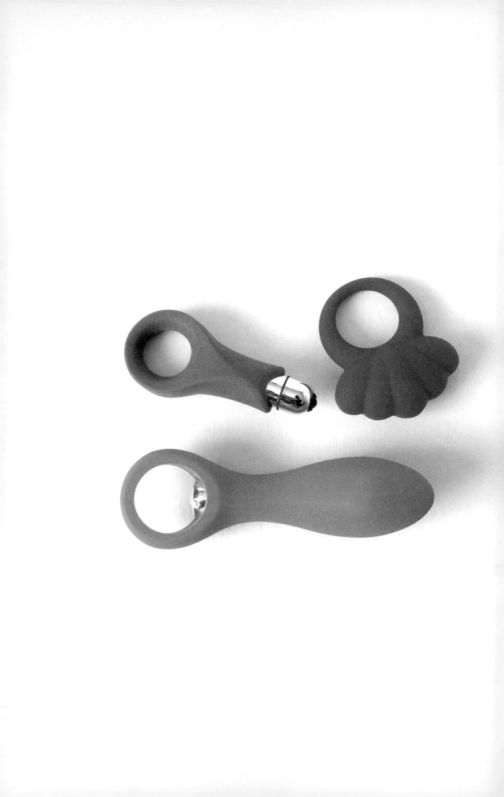

55

Put a Ring on It

Sometimes it's difficult to incorporate toys into actual sexy times: they get in the way, they fall out, they roll away, and so on, all of which ruins the mood, at least temporarily. Sometimes you just need a tool that was made for the job, and in those situations, you need a cock ring. Cock rings are as simple as they sound: it's just a ring that goes around a penis, and when you turn it on it vibrates. They come in stretchy material that you can loop around your partner's penis so that the toy stays in place, right at the base of his dick. And when you turn it on, you end up with the best of both worlds: a real live penis that vibrates as he fucks you! Plus, he gets to enjoy the buzz, too. This toy works in an endless number of positions, but you'll have better luck if you stick to girl-on-top, or other positions where the vibrating pack is right up against her clitoris.

56

More Ring Fun

Cock rings are a good time, and they are really convenient for couple's play! There are many different styles you can try to liven up your lovemaking. Some "couple's rings" as they are also called have an extra vibrating bit that extends out from the ring for extra stimulation. Turn the toy so that the extra piece is on top of his penis to stimulate your clitoris while he's fucking you, or rotate it the other way so that it sticks out from beneath his cock if you want some back door buzzing while you ride him. Different attachments create different sensations, and some toys come with different textures to add another level of touch to your play. Try different positions to get the whole effect!

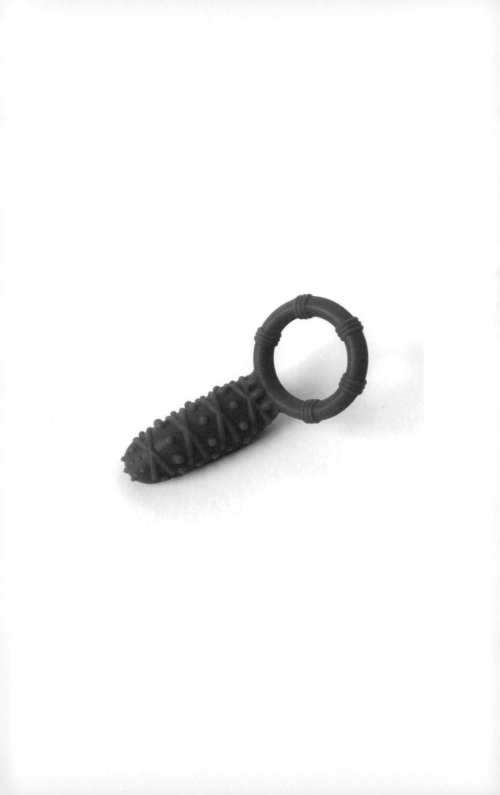

57

Reach Out and Touch Someone

If your partner is away or you're in a long-distance relationship, you can still heat things up with your vibe, you just need a little technological help! You can use your favorite video chat program to put on your own sexy show. Pick out your favorite vibe and get comfortable, and put your computer or webcam where he can see you. Then, use your hands and your toy to play! Let him give you instructions and ask questions. Narrate your movements and tell your partner exactly how it feels as you pleasure yourself! Make this game your own: you can make up a story as you go, and play out a scene. Or, you can just tell each other exactly what you want to do next time you're together.

58

Vibrator Races

So, good sex is not about coming fastest, but sometimes you just need a release, and you want it now. So why not make a game with your partner and see who can ride their toy to the finish line first? Start by having both of you pick your favorite toy and get comfy. Once you get going, you can tease one another, distract your partner, and turn them on! Make your own rules: can you just look and not touch each other? Can you talk, or is it gasps and grunts only? You get to decide exactly how you want to play. Decide on end game rules as well: if you declare the first to come the winner of the game, they get to decide how to finish their partner off! If you say the winner is whoever lasts the longest, then the loser is responsible for helping the winner get off however they want!

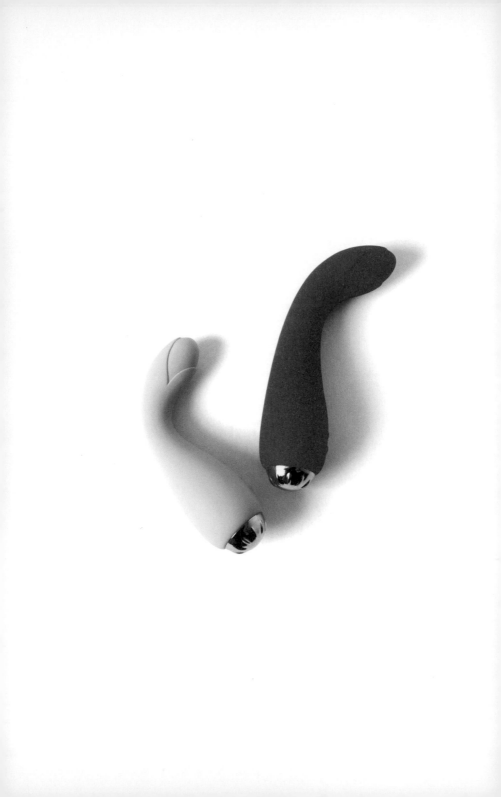

59

Vibrator Trivia

This game works best with a vibrator with a remote control, so that your partner can control it while you hold it in place. It plays like a regular game of trivia, but with a shocking penalty for wrong answers. First you'll need trivia questions, which you can pull from an old trivia board game, or off the internet, or you can come up with your own sexy questions! Once you have all of your props, find a place where you can recline comfortably, and hold your vibe in place. Start up your game and have your partner ask the first question! The penalty for one wrong answer is a short jolt, but if you keep getting the wrong answer, the penalty increases by one second for every question you've gotten wrong. For the last round, kick it up to the next level! Set the vibe to a low buzz to begin with. Then, as you go through the round, every time you get a question wrong, the vibe's intensity is turned up another notch. The distracting sensations make it harder to answer correctly, so you have to pay attention!

If you have more than one remote-controlled vibe, you can make this a head-to-head contest! You can follow the same rules as the Vibrator Races game, and let whoever holds out longest choose how he or she wants to finish the night!

60

The Counting Game

This is another game where you have to try and keep your concentration while your partner does their best to distract you! You can make this game as easy or as hard as you like. For the easy rules, you just have to count, slowly, as your partner stimulates you with a vibrator. If you miss a number, your partner gets to up the intensity of the toy and you start all over. You can simply count as your partner plays, or you can set the game up so that your partner continually pulses the vibe, and you count the pulses as he goes. He can try to make you slip up by changing his rhythm and speeding up or going very slow. If you like math and want to make this game harder, count up by twos, threes, or whatever integer you think is challenging enough for you. The game is over when you get to 100, or when you come. Then you can switch places for round two!

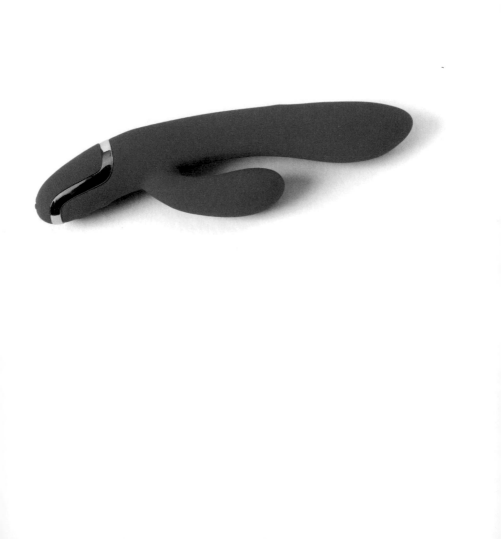

6d

Door Number One

Do you have so many toys you don't know which to play with?
Here's a hot game to make it easy. Get a piece of paper and
make two lists numbered one through six. Assign a body part to
each number, and then assign a different toy from your arsenal
for the other set of six. If you have fewer than six toys you can
double up or get creative, like listing hands and mouth as
other "toy" options. If you have more than six toys, you'll have
to choose your favorites, or use additional dice! Once you're
ready, take turns playing the game. Roll the dice first to see
which toy you use, then again to see where you get to use it!
You can set a timer if you want to play for a while before moving
to the next round, where your partner gets to try his luck! Or
you can up the ante and make a round last until you come
before you're allowed to switch!

62

Vibrator Merry-Go-Round

This game's a fun one for couples with a good collection of toys! Tired of always using the same tool to get the job done? Why not take a whirlwind tour through all of your favorite toys, even the ones you haven't dug out in a while! The point of this game is to try everything once. Line up your toys, and then pick a word to use when you change rounds (I like to use the word "change!"). This game is a lot like the "timing" game in this section, except instead of switching places when the timer goes, you decide when you want to move on. Start with one person laying on the bed while the other partner pleasures them with one of the toys: the partner doing the pleasing gets to pick. When the partner on the bed has had enough, he or she says "change!" the partners trade places, and the person in charge gets to pick a new toy to tease their partner with. If you can make it all the way through, you both get to pick which toy to use to finish off your tryst: if only one partner lasts the whole game, he or she gets to pick unilaterally.

63

Inside Reading

Reading sexy stories by yourself is hot. Reading sexy stories with a partner brings another kind of bliss. It isn't until you read these steamy tales while someone wields a vibrator that you have reached Nirvana. Choose an excerpt or a short erotica story neither of you have read that you know will get you both going. Start reading slowly, getting you and your partner into a sultry state of mind so that you both want a little more. Give him control of the vibrator as you work your way into the reading. He should tease you slowly, working his way along your sexiest spots and running his hands along your body. Keep the tantric approach as you read by maintaining your composure as long as you can, reading fluidly. As he eases the vibrator into you, varying his pace and the power level, it will become more and more difficult to remember what you were doing. Fight it! See how far you can get into the reading—and the vibrating—before you go over the edge. This will be amazing for you, and incredibly sexy for him.

64

Something Up Your Sleeve

No, a dick sleeve is not formal attire for your penis, although when you do use one to "dress up," you're in for a hell of a special occasion. Penis sleeves are like the next level of cock ring: they consist of flexible tubes that you slide over your dick to create new sensations when you're having sex. Vibrating sleeves come in many models with different textures and add-ons, all to give you a wild ride. These toys are often ribbed on the inside, to give him an extra boost! You can play with this toy in any position: with her on top she can groove and move her hips to savor the sensations. Try a deeper position, like with her feet on your shoulders, to enjoy the full length of his thrusts.

65

Good Timing

This game is designed to drive you wild—and to make you take turns! All you need is a timer and your favorite vibes. Each partner gets 30 seconds to use the vibe on their partner and try to really drive them crazy before the timer goes and the partners switch. You take turns teasing and pleasing one another and trying not to come too soon. The game is over if either partner either comes or begs to come. Whichever partner manages to last the longest is the "winner," and the other must finish them off however the winner decides. Make up your own end game rules, and see how many rounds you can last!

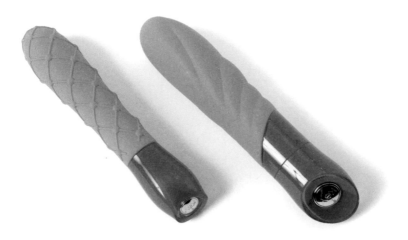

66

Sex Toy Hide and Seek

This was the ultimate game to play as a child, and it is even more fun with an adult twist! Hide different sex toys around the house and tell your partner to go find them. Make each of the toy selections unique, so that every time you move on to a new toy it is an entirely new sensation. Tuck a riding crop behind a doorway, hang a vibrating cock ring on a hook in the bathroom, or stow a rabbit vibrator in a coat pocket. Make it more exciting by removing the batteries to each of the vibe toys and force your partner seek those out too! The thrill of having a sexy toy but needing to find a way to turn it on will make the main event all the more exhilarating!

67

Pick a Card, Any Card

Strip poker is an enormous time suck when you could be spending your time with more enticing kinds of sucking. Skip the rules and regulations of a full poker game and instead set out a deck of cards for you and your partner. Assign tasks for each suit, like oral for hearts, BDSM toys for clubs, bullet or egg vibrators for spades, and your favorite vibrator for diamonds. If you want to get even more involved, assign specific tasks to each card, like seven-second vibrations for a 7 of diamonds, or cunnilingus with a bullet vibrator for the queen of hearts.

68

Quiet Seduction

If you are a vocal lover, sometimes keeping it quiet can be a daunting task. While in the throes with your partner, make a rule to have no sounds other than the sexy hum of the toy being used. No moans, no sighs, and especially no exclamations of "yes!" or "fuck me!" allowed. If you or your partner breaks the rules, the vibrator gets put away for sixty seconds and the offender gets teased everywhere but the hot spot. The inability to speak adds an extra level of earnestness and longing for pleasure and release, which will magnify the feeling of arousal and lead to an earth-shattering O.

69

Two Become One

Sex toys are super fun and erotic, but they can also be intimate. Using either a vibrating cock ring or a small vibrating toy, sit facing your partner with your legs wrapped around each other, as if cross-legged. If you are using a small toy that is not a cock ring, put it in before putting *him* in. With the vibe running, start with slow penetration, wrapping your arms around each other and making direct eye contact. Ease in and out, but not too quickly—you should both be concentrating on maintaining eye contact while feeling the gradual buildup of the vibrating sensations that connect you. By not breaking your gaze, you and your partner will feel the intensity of the passion between you and bring you to the pleasure pinnacle in tandem.

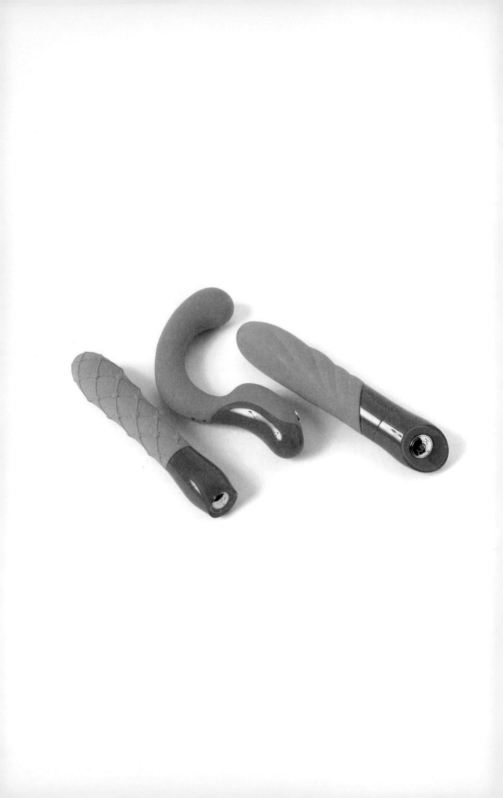

70

Mix and Match

Different toys can give you dramatically different sensations, even more so if you try more than one at once! Take a look at your collection and see what toys play well together. Try pairing toys with a specific use with toys you can use all over: like when you're using your vibrating butt plug, pull out your ring vibe so you can stimulate your nipples, clitoris, and other sensitive areas while the plug buzzes away. If you're playing with a wand vibe, you might want your vibrating bullets for internal stimulation. You can even mix and match when you're playing with a partner: try picking out one or two toys each, then take turns trying different combinations.

71

Perfect Stranger

Let's face it—when you have known someone for a long time, it becomes harder and harder to find something new to get you wet, hot, and bothered in no time at all. While you know exactly how to please your lover, it may just not have the same sizzle as when you first started dating. In this scenario, pretend you do not know one another. This could mean dressing up in outfits, introducing yourselves with different names, or both showing up at a bar you have never been to and locking eyes from across the room. By acting like you don't know each other, you have more freedom to entice and tease in ways you have never done before, or get naughty and try things you would not normally suggest. Tie in a traditional vibrator and let it tease places you have never wandered. Try something kinky, like vibrating nipple clamps and experiment like you have never done before. Be strangers in the night until you have satisfied your daring desires!

Sensation Play and BDSM

Introduction

Sensation play is the act of adding or removing different elements into your love sessions to intensify your senses. This can include toying with hot and cold temperatures, vibing with music, or even adding pain to your repertoire. If you want to take your vibrations to the next level, give your naughty routine a healthy smack with some tried and true BDSM techniques. BDSM—or *Bondage, Domination, Sadism, and Masochism*—is not for the faint of heart. For safety reasons, it is best to perform any BDSM techniques with a trusted partner—never alone. While intense BDSM can incorporate subservience and pain, you should never take part in these techniques if you do not feel comfortable, and always have a safe word for when you or your partner would like to stop. When performed with a partner you trust, BDSM *and* vibrations can be a mind-blowingly erotic addition to your sexual catalogue.

72

Tie Me and Tease Me

There is nothing sexier than seeing what you want and having to fight for it in the bedroom. Whether you are doing the tying up or you are the one strapped to the bed, chair, or elaborate bondage furniture, it is going to be hot. There are a few important rules before you engage in bondage play. A partner should never be left alone, bindings should never be so tight that they cut off circulation, and you should always have a pair of scissors handy in case you need to get loose in the event of an emergency or interruption. If you plan on putting weight or pressure on the bindings, make sure to evenly distribute the weight by tying more than one point along the limb. Once you have all of these things figured out, it is time to get tied and teased!

If you are the one in control and you have tied your partner up, experience your position of power to the fullest by doing lots of teasing! Kiss and tease in all of the sexiest zones, from the neck, chest, wrists, and along the beltline. Get your favorite vibrator revving, and drag it slowly along the inside of the legs, but delay directly hitting the sweet spot. Watch your partner get riled up and beg for more while you tease and play! The ropes, ties, or other bindings will keep your partner restrained and make the temptation even more intense. Incorporating vibrations with enticing restraints will take this sexy session to new heights!

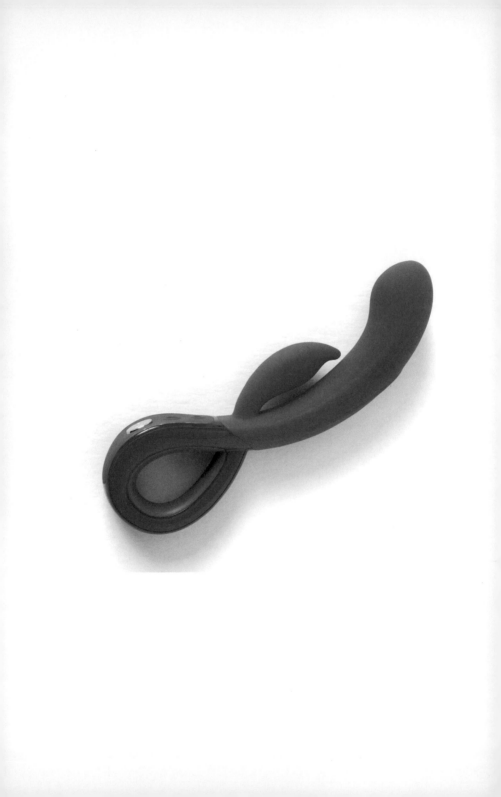

73

Arrest Warrant

Be naughty, be the bad cop! With a pair of fuzzy handcuffs, restrain your criminal for a little corporal punishment. With either two sets of handcuffs attached to each hand and a corresponding bedpost, or one set of handcuffs restraining just the arms, use your vibrator as a policeman's baton and dole out some sentences! (Just remember, while a good smack with a vibrator can get you and your partner feeling hot and kinky, never hit areas like the head, torso, or spine to avoid serious injury.) While your prisoner is helpless, hot, and bothered, use the vibrator to play good cop and bad cop. If your partner has been naughty, give him a good paddle to the ass and show him who is in charge. If he has been very good, use the vibrator on him in places that will make him super hot. Switch back and forth to keep both of your tantric tempos way up until you are ready to give in to each other.

74

Polar Vibes

Just because it is cold does not mean it can't be hot. Incorporating sensation play with temperatures is an intense way to ramp up your passionate playtime. Test your limits with an ice massager, which combines erotic vibrations with an enticing chill. These massagers are orb-like in shape, so they are meant for body massaging, rather than insertion. Some ice enthusiasts recommend experimenting with ice dildos, but this can be dangerous because you can cool down your core body temperature too quickly. The ice massagers bring in the excitement without any of the drawbacks, and they won't melt into a puddle like ice cubes! The only preparation is to allow for freezing time once you have filled the orb with water. Whether you play alone or play with a partner, bring the massager along sensitive areas like the nipples, inside of the arms, inner thighs, beltline and sides of the torso. The vibrations and the cold chill will have you covered in goose bumps and writhing in pleasure. After you have taken all you can handle, bring the ice massager to your hot spot and let the amazing sensation surprise you. The intensity of the cold and the vibrations will bring your orgasm to an entirely new place!

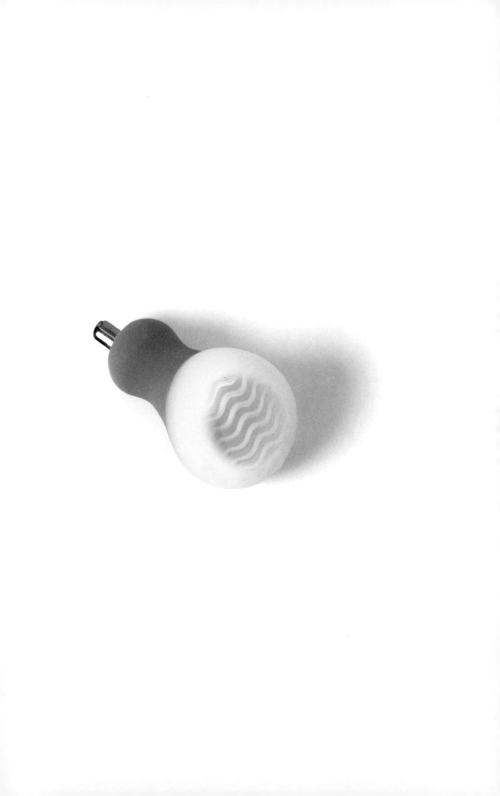

75

Power Yoga

If you are not familiar with yoga, it's time to get in tune with your body, mind, and pleasure zone. Yoga helps you relax, strengthen and stretch your body, and concentrate on your inner spirit. By focusing on the movements of your body and the muscles you are using in each pose, you are able to brush away the concerns and stressors from your life that weigh you down. While traditional yoga is spiritually and physically satisfying on its own, the investment in your body as you transition your yoga poses can easily align with your sexuality. Slide your favorite small vibrator inside you, or secure a large vibrator shaft with a suction cup base to the mat or floor. As you transition through each pose, pause by lowering yourself onto the rotating or vibrating shaft and peacefully accepting the pleasure. When you become overwhelmed with the physical intensity of the yoga poses and vibrating bliss, your calming yoga experience may end with some hot aerobics to get you to your amazing climax!

76

Mirror, Mirror

The slow hum or the fast buzz of your vibrator should definitely get you going, but vibrations play should be an experience that overwhelms the senses, and not just touch. Set yourself up in front of a mirror and take in the image of yourself and how sexy you look. Rub your hands along your body and begin to tease yourself. Keep the mirror in place and gently begin to incorporate the vibrator into your mirror time. Get up close and personal with your body and the mirror, watch yourself slide the vibrator in and out, witnessing how your body reacts to the enticing buzz and motions of the toy. Flushed cheeks and rosy curves are super sexy, so turn yourself on! The visual stimulation of being able to see how you look and feel while you are close to coming will add a whole new thrill to your repertoire!

77

Nipple Nympho

For the woman who loves extra attention on her breasts and nipples, there is more to be explored! Try incorporating vibrating breast massager into your solo play or couple's foreplay to add a little spice to your routine. These soft, jelly-like massagers cup around the nipple and breast and contain vibrating nubs on each cup. While this toy is super fun, the massagers can sometimes fall out of place or unstick. If they do, consider using skin-safe adhesive (like one you would use for eyelash extensions) so that you can get naughty without worrying about wardrobe malfunctions. This fun massager sends sultry vibrations to tickle your nipples to make them hard, tantalize the senses, and get you hot and ready for more.

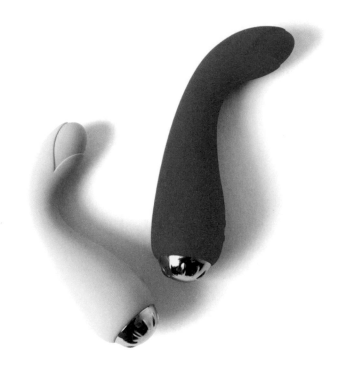

78

Tantalizing Tingles

Vibrators are meant to intensify your passionate playtime, but even a vibrator can use a little extra pizzazz. An amazing way to add to the pleasure your vibrator provides is by incorporating tingly body lubricant. Rub yourself and your vibrator down with a minty gel or a peppermint lubricant specifically designed for sexy play. The gentle tingle will invigorate your senses and send a cooling effect to your hot spots. The extra awakening will help you feel every inch of the hard shaft inside you and propel the hum of the vibrations against your most sensitive areas to a new level. The intensity of the extra sensations will be an exhilarating way to make your traditional vibe session even better!

79

Think Outside the Box

Get into the mood without ever touching your lady bits! Okay, so maybe you will want to touch them *eventually*, but try focusing your attentions on every part of you except for your clitoris and vaginal area to send you into a total-body sexual Zen. Turn your vibrator on to a low speed and caress all of your erogenous zones, from the inside of your arms, to the side of your torso, over your breasts and inside your legs. Let the hum of the toy lull you into sexual euphoria and intensify your arousal. Massaging every part of your body will perk your senses and make you hyper aware of the aching pleasure between your legs! Clench your kegel muscles while you caress your body with the buzzing vibes, and if you immerse yourself deeply enough into the sensations running through your body, you may even be able to come without ever bringing the vibrator to your pussy.

80

Mystery Vibes

While many forms of sensation play revolve around *adding* a sensation to a given method of pleasuring, using a blindfold works in the opposite way by removing the sense of sight. With the inability to see what your partner is doing, your other senses, especially hearing and touch, are magnified. This intensity makes for a heart-pounding sexy session because you never know where you will be touched next! Make your vibe play all the more exciting by incorporating a blindfold and playing a guessing game. Incorporate multiple vibrators and pleasure your partner (or be pleasured) with each one. Without touching the toy, you or your partner should guess the kind of vibrator that is being used. Guessing the method of choice will give you extra focus on the sensations at hand, the feel of their rhythm, firmness, or how aroused you become!

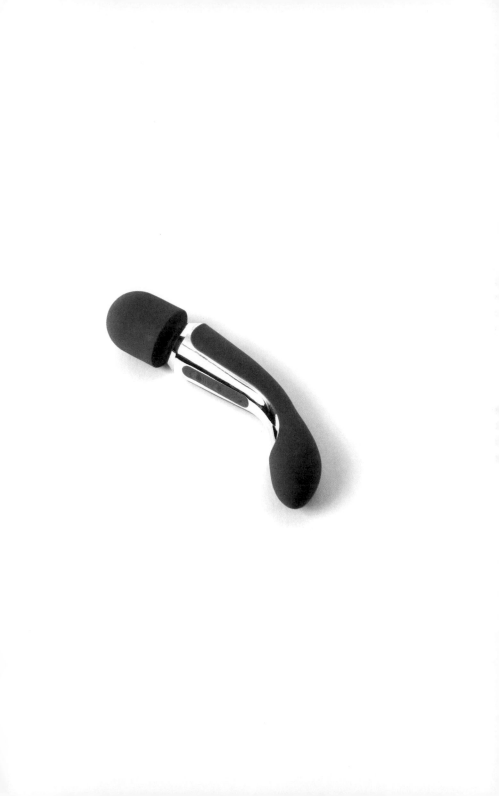

81

Conductor's Baton

With this blindfolding technique, the one who is in the dark has all the power! Like a conductor at a symphony, lie down blindfolded and instruct your skilled musician. Tell him where to go and conduct how fast the rhythm should be or how hard he should play. The blindfold is an exciting way to see if your music-maker follows your lead, or brings you to new places if he prefers to go off on a solo. This electrifying approach to blindfolding combines the best of both worlds in sensation play—the blindfolding process allows you to feel submissive and at the will of your lover, but your role as conductor asserts your dominance and allows you to dictate just how you want to be pleased!

82

Savasana

Savasana is a still pose often used at the end of a yoga session to relax your body and refresh your spirit. After an hour or more of stretching your body through yoga, *savasana* is a peaceful position where you lie flat with your arms and legs comfortably rested, allowing you to release all of the tension in your muscles. Apply this to your moments of bliss by lying down still. Relax your muscles and even out your breathing. Slide your vibrator into your pussy and turn it on the lowest setting. Put your hands at your sides and breathe in and out deeply, allowing your body to relax and take in the slow pulse of the toy. Do not clench your kegel muscles or move your pelvis in any way. Allow the vibrations to take you up a slow and steady incline to a sexual Nirvana.

83

Removable Showerheads and Waterproof Vibrators: Greater or Greatest?

It's time for a competition between the most satisfying accidental sex toy and the most satisfying invented one! Gone are the days of lifting your leg high against the shower wall to feel some water pressure on your lady bits, risking serious slip-and-fall injuries! Removable showerheads are the vagina's greatest aqua ally. Bring your waterproof vibrator into the shower and put it to the test against the showerhead. Massage your clitoris with the pulsing water, and insert the humming vibrator into your wet and ready pussy. Increase the settings on the shower head to send a steady pulse to your love nub, or let it spray widely to tantalize your whole hot spot. Clench your muscles to the rhythm of the vibrator while you let the pressure build from all angles. Let the two work in unison and bring you to a sexual peak over and over again!

84

Get into Hot Water

One of the greatest parts of pleasuring yourself in the shower is the warmth of the water. Try starting out with a cold or lukewarm shower while getting hot with your vibrator. (Never bring sex toys into the water that are not explicitly waterproof.) Angle the spray of the water toward your pussy and ride your sex toy slowly. The cool water will get your tits firm and tingly and awake your body's senses. Gradually increase the temperature, warming the shower so that your body relaxes. Move the vibrator in and out of your pussy and let yourself feel the warmth of the shower spray. Angling the water directly on your clitoris (if you do not have a removable showerhead, you will have to get a little flexible and stretch your legs), turn the water up hot (not scalding!) so that the intense heat increases the arousing sensations of the vibrator and the pressure on your clitoris. The hot water against you will make your orgasm all the more satisfying!

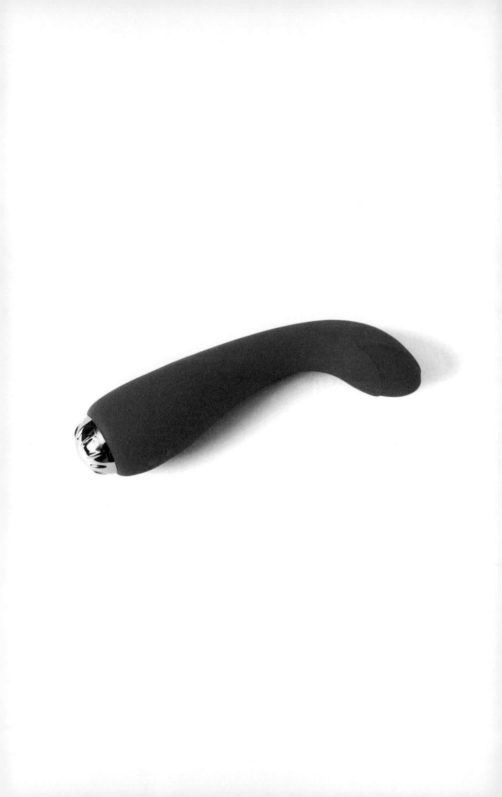

85

Bubble Bath Bliss

The only thing more sensual than a bubble bath is a bubble bath with sex toys! Many vibrators are designed to be waterproof specifically for this purpose, so find one that really turns you on. Set your bathroom up to be an area of complete relaxation. Turn on tranquil music, light candles, and add scented bath gels to the steamy water. Allow yourself to relax in the tub, letting the warmth lull you into a peaceful state. Get turned on by turning on your vibrator and easing it into you. Take in the scents of the bath gels and calming light from the candles, and slowly pleasure your pussy with the hum of the toy. Let out moans and hear the ecstasy in your own voice as the bliss starts to overwhelm you. Draw out your pleasure for a long, sensual bath so that your body is completely relaxed and ready for when you finally let yourself come.

86

In Your Hot Seat

Lady parts are not the only areas that get aroused from a hot water massage. While in the shower, face away from the spray and bend forward to allow the water to pound against your backside. From the inside of your thighs, to your cheeks, to in between, your bum is one of the most sensitive areas of your whole body. Even if you are not partial to anal stimulation, the hot water against this sensitive naughty zone is a powerful hint to your other pleasure hubs that erotic enjoyment is on its way. Use your waterproof vibrator to entice your clitoris and fuck your pussy while the hot water stimulates your back end. This is a fun way to feel a little dirty while getting clean!

87

Waterfall

Water pressure and vibrations are every woman's allies. Draw half a bubble bath so that the water is not too high and lie down in the tub. Scoot your bum to the front of the tub by the faucet, letting your legs rest to the side or lie in an L position with them up against the wall. Make sure the water keeps you warm but is not so high that your face is underwater. Bring a vibrator with a rotating head in with you and slide it inside you so that it massages deep inside your vagina and stimulates your g-spot. Turn the faucet on full blast so that it sends a direct stream to your clitoris, sending a hard, intense pressure waterfall to launch you in to ecstasy. The powerful flow of water will overwhelm your pleasure hub and, in tandem with the massager inside you, will bring you to a full-body, mind-blowing orgasm.

88

Roooxanne

Get saucy and sensual to the beat of music, but add this extra step. Choose a song that you find particularly enticing or gets you revved up, preferably if it has a lot of repetition in its lyrics. Select a word or a particular phrase that comes up in the song a lot. Keep your vibrator in neutral until each time you hear this word or phrase, and then turn the vibrator on full throttle. This trick will give you quick spurts of erotic excitement and maintain a heightened level of desire. If you want to keep going, just put the song on repeat!

89

Hot Hot Heat

Turn up the heat on your playtime by incorporating hot oils and warming lubricants. Massage your body with warm oil to feel slippery and sexy. The warmth will tingle against your skin and the oil will make you feel primed and ready for some penetrative vibrations. Rub your whole body, from your breasts, to your sides, to the insides of your legs and all around your sexy zone. Use warming lubricants over the vibrator shaft; making sure it is slick as you ease it inside you. The heat from the lubricant will send radiating pleasure inside you that will make your eventual orgasm feel like it is practically glowing.

90

Spankalicious

Sometimes spanking is to show who is the Dom and who is the Sub during kinky playtime. Other times, it is more of a natural reaction, as in, "Holy shit, this feels so good, I need to smack something!" Whichever way you like to get red in the cheeks, try it with some sensory overload. Using a vibrating cock ring for him or a vibrating egg for her, turn on the naughty by letting the vibes roll. While the slow vibrations and subtle hum to your sweet spots get you primed, get feisty, too! Be the spanker or the spankee and add some spice to your scenario. Use an open palm and leave a nice red handprint, or purchase a kinky spanking paddle that leave verbal imprints like "FUCK ME" and "KINKY." Be nice and get a fuzzy paddle to soften the blow. Whichever your fancy, the tantric tango between the vibrations and a little painful pleasure will offer you a sex romp you will feel long after you've come!

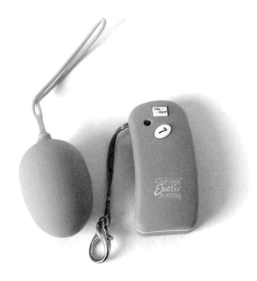

91

Power Play

Getting turned on with your partner when you think you might get caught is super sexy, but see what happens when only he has access to the Off button. The next time you are out on the town, insert your remote-controlled egg or bullet and give him the switch. He gets all the control while you sit tight, waiting for that buzz of pleasure. As you spend your night out at a show, dinner, or huddled close at a packed bar, the anticipation of a little surprise ecstasy will get you both in a hot vibe. He can choose to start off slowly, with small spurts of light vibrations to have you inching your way to a mind-blowing orgasm. If he thinks you have been a little naughty, he can skip the foreplay and give you full power doses to have you climaxing at every pause in the conversation. Whether he takes the whole evening to get you worked up, or constantly throws you over the edge while you try to order your drinks, this will be one evening you will love to lose control!

Pleasure for Your Caboose

Butt Stuff Safety

Using toys for anal play can be a really fun and exciting experience for you and your partner, but there are a few rules to follow to make sure you have a safe and stress-free experience.

What Goes in Must Come Out

The most important rule for butt play is that you shouldn't put anything in anyone's ass unless you're sure you can get it back out. Someone once said to me that "a vagina's a cul-de-sac, but your ass is a freeway!" which is one of the strangest non-sequiturs I've ever heard but is also a helpful reminder that while the vagina is a closed system with no way for a toy to get "lost," your ass is not, and a "lost" toy can create serious medical issues. To stay safe, only use toys that are sold explicitly for anal play, and make sure that your toys have a base that is thicker than the rest of the toy so that they cannot accidentally be inserted all the way.

No Sharp Edges

You shouldn't have trouble with this if you follow the rules and only use toys intended for anal play, but it's worth repeating: the skin inside your ass is sensitive and delicate, so make sure any toy you use is smooth and has no sharp edges.

Use Lube

Butts don't make their own lube like vaginas sometimes do, so you're going to need a good personal lubricant to enjoy yourself. Water-based lube is a good bet, since it's the only kind safe for use with condoms and all sex toy materials. Using oil or other petroleum-based lubes (like petroleum jelly) can damage some toys and degrade condoms. This goes for natural oil lubes like coconut oil, as well.

Keep It Clean

It's important to clean your toys before and after you use them to keep them squeaky clean, and this is especially true for anal toys, which can carry germs that can make you sick. The easiest way to keep toys clean is to use a condom: when you're done you can just peel it off and you're set! You can also use a female condom for this purpose, which works just as well to prevent mess, and may even be more comfortable, but they are also potentially less effective at preventing transmission of STDs, so if this is a concern for you, stick with the male condom.

Even if you are using a condom, you should clean your toys before and after play, with some soap and hot water. You should make sure your anal toys are made out of a nonporous material that is easily sterilized, like silicone, borosilicate glass, and stainless steel. Stay away from jelly and rubber, which are much more difficult to keep clean.

It Shouldn't Hurt

It is really important to remember when engaging in anal play that if it hurts, you are doing something wrong. Do not "tough it out," and stay away from numbing lubes, because if it is hurting, you may be doing damage and the pain is there to tell you to stop what you are doing! If you take it slow, use plenty of lube, and stop whenever it becomes uncomfortable, you should have a good experience!

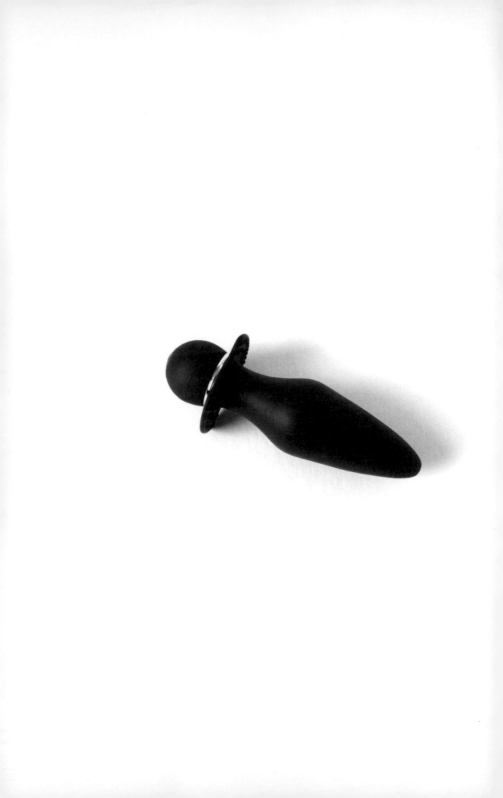

92

Plug It In

Vibrating butt plugs are fun for anal play beginners and long time fans alike! You can get butt plugs in just about any size or shape you want. Some plugs come in sets ranging in size, which are made to help you get used to larger plugs and stimulators. Beginner plugs are usually smaller and are often called "trainer" plugs. Check out the tips on page 140 to help you pick out a safe toy.

You can play with a butt plug by yourself, or play with your partner! First, get warmed up: anal play works best when you're relaxed and super turned on. Make out with your partner, masturbate, maybe play with a vibrator, and get yourself revved up before you try the plug. When you're ready, lube up the toy and slowly and gently slide it into your ass. If you're playing with your partner, it can be fun to grind against them as you slide yourself onto the plug. Keep going until the larger part of the plug is inside you and the wide base is sitting at the outside of your asshole. Then, turn on the plug and experience the new sensation! Men and women can both enjoy playing with butt plugs: men especially can get a special thrill out of the toy, which stimulates their prostate, the sensitive gland that some people call the "male g-spot."

93

Oral and Butt Plug

Oral sex and back door stimulation is a winning combo for both partners, so try this during foreplay, or as the main course! Start by going down on your partner, then as things get hot and heavy, use your fingers to gently circle their asshole. Use your fingers to add lube (and try not to get lube in your mouth), and then slowly insert the plug. Don't slow down or pause your oral ministrations, if you can help it! Turn on the plug and enjoy the fireworks! Use a hand or other convenient body part to brace the plug if your partner wants to grind against it.

If your partner is a dude, pay extra attention to his cock as you're putting in the plug, and try out alternating between slow deep throating and faster pumping strokes. Play with his balls to add to the total overwhelming mix of sensations!

If your partner is a lady, make sure to concentrate on her clitoris, and alternate your speed and technique. Slide your fingers inside of her and stroke her g-spot: follow her lead and let her grind against you and set her own tempo.

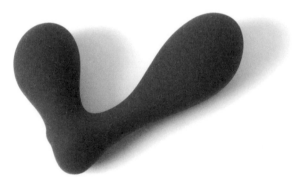

94

Butt Plug Double Penetration

Double penetration is a winning move in the pornos, and now you can try it in the comfort of your own home! Vibrating butt plugs work great for this position, because unlike other toys, they stay put. You can swing this move in a couple different positions, so try a few to find out what works best for you! If your man is a little bigger, girl-on-top may be your best bet: once the butt plug toy is in place, have your partner help you turn it on. Then climb on top and slowly slide him into you, taking time to get used to the deep, rumbly full feeling. In Cowgirl or reverse Cowgirl, you'll have the most control over the speed and depth of his thrusts. Or for a wilder ride, try it doggy style! Using a butt plug, you might find that your regular doggy style angle doesn't work: in this case, use a pillow under your hips to help you get the right fit, and adjust by moving from resting on your hands and knees to resting on your elbow and knees, or lying with your upper body on the bed. This position is much more butt-centric, and it will give your partner a great view as you're going at it! Plus your partner will be free to readjust the toy or just slap that ass.

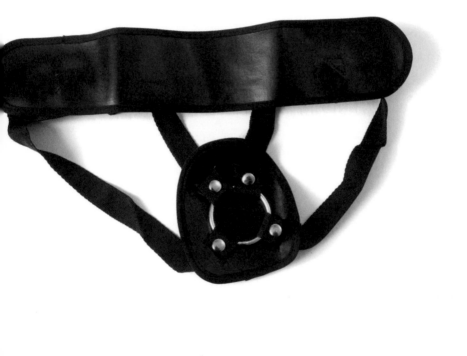

95

Pegging for Dummies

Pegging sounds like it's some kind of cute, old-fashioned game, or maybe a version of Plinko. In actuality, it is the term for when a woman uses a strap on device to penetrate and stimulate her partner. It is a fun way to switch up roles in the bedroom, and it looks sexy as fuck. If you've graduated past the vibrating butt plugs, pegging is a must-try next step.

The most basic vibrating strap on rigs consists of a vibrating dildo strapped to a harness-contraption you secure around your hips and waist. Make sure the straps are tight enough so that you can effectively wield your newfound phallus, and retighten them when you get into position. As with the other butt toys, it's best to get revved up before you start. When your partner is ready, have him get into whatever position is most comfortable: you can have him lay back and prop his hips up on a pillow and take him from the front, like a modified missionary, or bend him over the side of the bed in the more traditional doggy style. Give him a reach-around, and stroke him with your hands as you move, or hold on to his hips, and have him give you a show.

You also have a few options for working a bit of her pleasure into pegging play. There are harnesses that include a strategically placed vibrator for her, or you can make your own rig by tucking your own vibrator into the straps, or better yet, inserting a vibrating bullet into your vagina and tucking the remote into your harness. There are also "strapless strap-ons," a kind of dual vibrator that you hold in place with your vagina while you use the other end to fuck your partner.

96

Bead It

Anal beads are a fun addition to any sex toy ensemble, and like most anal toys, they'll work for men and women—just about anyone with a butt, really. Anal beads consist of several round beads strung together on a thick sturdy string of some kind. Many beginner sets come with graduated beads, meaning they start small on one end of the strand and get larger as you move toward the end. Some anal beads, especially many of the vibrating types, also come in a more "stick-like" version, where the beads are attached to a soft flexible material, making it more like a bulbous stick than a string of beads, but this makes the toy a bit easier to use, and much easier to vibrate. Vibrating anal beads are set up so that the vibrations run through the entire toy, so you can get a buzz even if you're using "just the tip." Play with your anal beads by lubing them up and inserting the beads into you or your partner's butt one by one. You don't need to insert the whole toy, just as much as you feel comfortable with! Once the beads are inserted, move around a bit: the beads move, too, and create all new sensations, especially with the extra jolt from the vibrations!

Another neat trick with anal beads is that they feel good going in and coming back out: some people enjoy the sensation of having the beads pulled out all at once as they climax. Test this out and see how it feels, but go slow!

Try inserting anal beads before sex to double your sensations! Try this out in a position where your partner can have access to the beads, so that he can move them around or try sliding them in and out as you play. If the beads are for you, doggy style is a good bet, and if it's his turn to play, try reverse cowgirl!

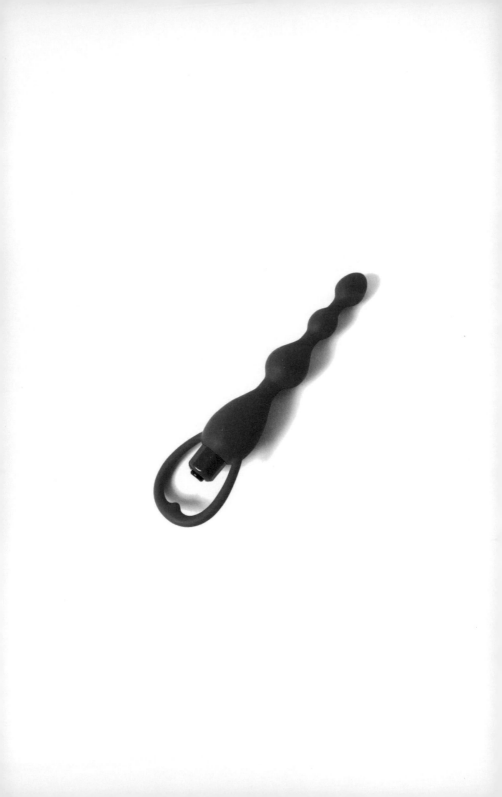

97

Pleasure in Your Hand

Anal T vibrators work a lot like butt plugs, except that they are easier to hold and use by hand than are butt plugs. These toys are usually built a lot like an egg vibrator, with the functional part attached to a controller by a long cord. The vibrating part itself is mostly shaped similar to a T: the "arms" of the T stick out at the base for easy handling, and to keep the toy safely wider at the base, to prevent you from accidentally losing it. These toys come in lots of different sizes, so you can find one that fits your style. Many of the models also have an angled shaft: these are specifically made for men, as the angled bit is used to stimulate his prostate.

> Small movements go a long way in butt play; so once the toy is in place, don't thrust with it. Instead, try a more gentle in and out movement, or rock the toy back and forth.

98

Vibrating Probes and Teasers

Anal toys come in lots of shapes and sizes, and while butt plugs and beads are about filling you up, there are other toys that explore the different kinds of sensations that come from anal play. Probes and teasers are usually slimmer than plugs, and are shaped like a phallus or a ribbed wand. Some models even let you bend and adjust them to give you just what you want. Since these toys are typically longer as well as thinner than plugs and other toys, they're a better choice for trying out more in-and-out sensations with butt play, and getting a feel for different textures and levels of penetration. You can use these on yourself or play with a friend, just take it slow!

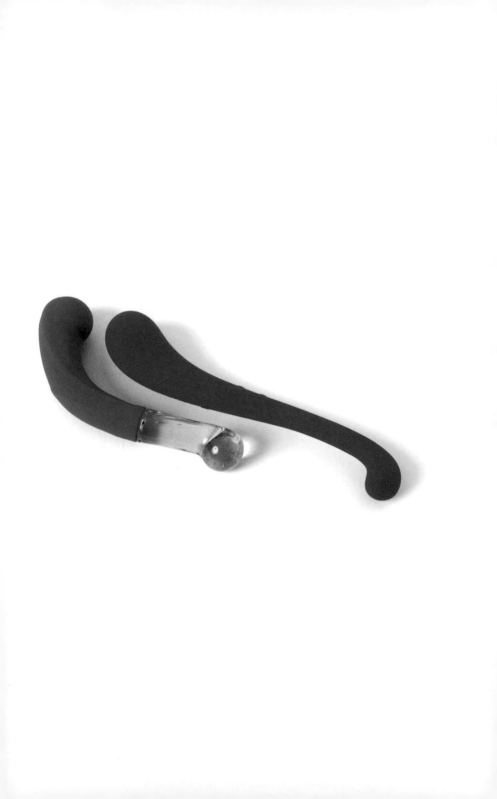

99

Pushing His Buttons

Butt stuff can be fun for both partners, but some men get a special thrill from anal play that stimulates their prostate. There are a bunch of toys on the market for just this purpose, and they can be used during solo play or during partner sex. As with any anal play, you start out with lube. Insert the toy comfortably, and then go to town! Keep up stimulation of his shaft and balls while you play with the vibe, and let him set the speed of the toy. Use both hands, and let him show you how he likes the toy to move. Strong in-and-out movements might not hit the spot: instead try smaller rocking movements to make the toy gently stroke his prostate. You'll definitely know when you get it right!

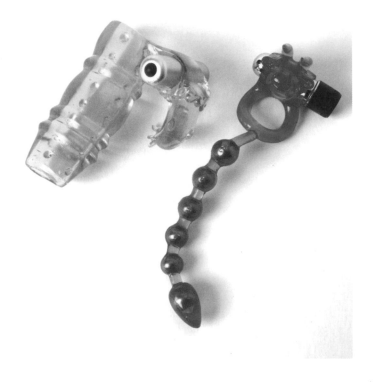

100

Beaded Buzz Ring

If a cock ring no longer excites you, and a vibrating ring is just another boring toy, then it's time to step in the arena with the sex ring pros. Introduce yourself to the vibrating cock ring and pleasure bead team! For his solo use or couples' pleasure, this mighty buzzer has a stretchy ring for him, a vibrating love nub for her, and a long gel rope of weighted beads that vibe in tandem with both. With a silky lubricant, slide the pleasure beads into your naughtiest spot while you ride him. You will be able to feel the buzz of the ring against your clitoris, and the humming intrigue of the beads from behind. Or since his back end is so sensitive, let him use the beads while you enjoy the clitoral stimulator on his shaft. If you like it from all angles, this can be an intense solo act for him, or a wild ride for two!

Erotica for Your Pleasure

JOJ

Joy Parties by Nicole Wilder

The warm shower water slithered its way down my body, over my firm breasts, hard nipples, tight abs and between my creamy, pink thighs. The heat made me quiver at first, before making me ache to touch myself. After lathering my hands with the lilac-scented shower gel, I let my slippery fingers run down my body languishing against the soft mounds of my breasts. As I squeezed each one, my nipples grew hard and ached for more. I massaged my large breasts, then brought one up to my lips and nibbled. Moments later, my right hand slid down my body and my legs spread slightly. I wanted, needed to touch the sweet, pink bulb inside. My mound was slippery and wet and fun to play with. I slipped my finger inside the lips to my aching clit. It was hard already as I began to circle around it. My other hand continued to massage my breasts and pinch and pull my nipples. As I grew more excited, I sat on the side of the tub under the flowing water. I spread my quivering thighs open, and let the water run over my clit.

I looked down to watch my hand squeeze my pussy, before dipping my finger deep inside myself. My hips moved up and down, meeting my disappearing fingers as I engaged more of them in the slippery fun. I loved watching me playing with myself, it excited me even more. My fingers came back into view, and with my left hand I opened my lips so I could see myself circle and wiggle my clit until I neared orgasm, then stop and squeeze the mound. I didn't want to come yet, it felt too good to want to stop.

When I thought I could continue to play again without coming too fast, I looked on the side of the tub where my little toy sat waiting to be used. I made it myself, an electric toothbrush that had great speed. I wrapped the end in a small nubby condom. The vibration of the tooth-brush and the nubby part of the condom drove my clit insane. I picked up the toy and leaned back a little, spreading my legs as wide as I could and ran the vibrating toothbrush over the lips of my pussy just to tease myself. I shook all over and moaned uncontrollably, it made me so horny that I knew I could have come in a few seconds, but I wanted to continue to hold off, so I could enjoy my favorite little pleasure toy. After spreading the lips of my pussy, I let the vibration run around my clit, dip inside me, then back around my clit.

A deep groan came from within my throat, and I nearly yelled as the vibration made me shake wildly. I wanted to come right away and yet, I wanted the sensation to last. Without thinking, I slipped it up inside my pussy as far as I could get it to go and moved it around in me, in circles, from side to side, in and out, anything I could think of to do with it. I jammed it hard into me and screamed in ecstasy, I could hear how wet I was even over the warm water that still ran over me.

"I need to come." I took the vibrator out of me and let it rest on my clit as hard as I could until entire body shook like I was convulsing. "Come!" I obeyed myself, the wetness of my pussy flowed freely from inside me. I could feel the warmth of it running down to my ass. I set my homemade vibrator down, and used my fingers to play in the wetness. It felt so good to rub it over my clit and down around my ass. Then I dipped my fingers deep inside myself bringing the wetness up to my nipples and coating them before bringing one of them to my lips to taste. I was so excited I hardly wanted it to stop, and yet, the quivering eventually subsided and my clit went back to normal.

"Wow!" I moaned. I finished my shower and naked I went into my bedroom. Still horny, I sat on the side of the bed, my legs spread wide, grabbed my smooth, plastic vibrator from the side drawer, turned it on and slid it into my still wet pussy. Staring between my legs, I rammed the vibrator in and out of myself like I was being wildly fucked. My hips swung up and down to meet it. "More, I need more." After a few more thrusts, I brought it out of myself to my clit and rested it on the most excited part of myself. "Come. Oh, please, come again." I needed it again more than ever, once just wasn't enough that day. In only a second, I started to quiver as my orgasm took over my mind and body. As I came back to reality, I slid the vibrator inside me and slowly moved it in and out to bring myself back down.

I was so happy for my toys. I loved sex toys. They were more fun with someone else, but when I didn't have another person to please me, at least I had my toys. With fifteen toys in my arsenal, I was never without a change of pace. It was almost an addiction for me. My partners loved my toys, loved to use them on me and loved watching me use them on myself.

Once I stopped shaking, I got dressed, went downstairs, and jumped on the Internet to see what was going on. I checked my e-mail, Facebook, bills, and then went to look on my favorite sex toy site to see what they had that was new. To my joy, they now had HERC! A giant-sized dildo that looked like it would be extremely fun and exciting to cram deep inside myself. I wondered how much of it would fit into me, but I knew no matter what, it would sure be fun to try it. I clicked the "add to cart" button to finish the order. I couldn't wait until it arrived at my house. Before getting out of the site, I saw a page that caught my eye.

"Sell fun toys to your friends. Make extra money while pleasing others." I continued to read and found out that I could sell these awesome, thrilling toys and make a little money while I did it. I thought about it, and I knew that I could make my marketing skills work for me. There had to be a way to make some big money selling something that I was addicted to. So I signed up to sell toys for the company, and put my marketing mind to work.

For my first party, I advertised to only friends and threw one of those stupid parties where people come to look at your items, buy a few, and leave. I only sold three. It wasn't until my parties became a little more wild that I sold a lot more.

My first thought was, who would want to buy my toys? Everyone loves sex. Everyone has a potential to love my toys. So my second thought was what could I do to get them to buy from me? Then it dawned on me. Let them try them there at the party. They would be able to try out the merchandise before they buy it.

My first wild party was all women. I advertised sexual demonstration of the toys. Twenty women showed up ready to try them out on themselves, me, and each other. I didn't know how it would turn out, but I was willing to do a lot to make my business work.

I came to the party dressed in a black bikini. I figured if I had to try out toys it would be the quickest way to undress. I laid out all the toys from giant dildos to edible panties. Once everyone quieted down I began to explain each one.

"Wow, I'd love to try that thing out," one woman said, pointing to a very large dildo called Gorge. "If I like it, I will buy it."

It was one of my most expensive toys. I took the dildo and walked over to her, and the rest of the women cheered.

"Show us how it's done," one lady said.

I put some lube on the toy and set it down while I slid off her panties and spread her legs. I licked one of my fingers and put it between her soft pink thighs. I wanted to make sure she was good and wet. She watched me, but I received no rejection. She moaned as I played with her clit, the other women either watched contently or cheered us on. I stuck two fingers well up inside her to find that she was already soaked.

Gorge was next to meet her sweet, little pussy. She spread her legs wide for me. I started out slow, and entered her a little at a time.

"Shove it in her," someone said. "Make her take it all."

She thrust her hips forward to take in more and then one of the other women joined me by playing with her breasts and pinching her nipple. She told my guinea pig, "Fuck the huge cock." She seemed only happy to do so, as I shoved it into her as deep as I could. She moaned loudly welcoming it, only a few thrusts into her wet canal, and she came.

"I will take it," she said, trembling wildly with Gorge still inside her.

"Can I try this one?" Some lady named Sue asked. It was a smooth plastic vibrator shaped like a cock without the detail.

"Absolutely," I told her. "Would you like me to show you a fun way to use it?"

"Yes, please," she said, tearing off her clothes, lying down and spreading her legs as the other women watched. Sue had a sweet, pink, shaven pussy and her lips were already swollen with excitement.

"I'm going to turn this one on so it vibrates, and bring it to your excited little clit like this," I said. I circled her clit as she squirmed with joy.

"Oh, my, more," she moaned. I moved it slightly into the wet hole to make the vibrator wet, so I could slip it deep into her pussy then back out. I thrust it into her several times, before bringing it out to hold it against her clit. I knew it would only take a moment for her to come.

"Make her come hard," a woman named Jan said, and I did. Sue yelled her orgasm as I reached up and pinched her nipple while she shook.

I looked over and the first woman was using another toy on the lady that helped me make her come, and she was really enjoying it.

"Dana, I see you eying that smooth vibrator Sue had, but try this one. It not only excites your clit, but tingles your ass at the same time," I told her.

"I'll help her with that," Robin said, and came over to her, getting her up on her hands and knees, and started to work on her. I watched for a moment to see Robin rubbing the woman's soft, excited mound, slapping her slightly, then moving her hand over her open pussy to play contently with her. I saw the glow of her wetness before Robin took the vibrator to thrust it into her, the little end at her ass. The woman being worked on played with her breasts, threw her head back and moaned loudly.

As the women with the toys enjoyed themselves, it became a feeding frenzy with the others. All the women picked their favorite toys and either used them on themselves or each other. It was such a great sight. Each of the women moved the toys in and out of their pussies or over their clits. Moans, and even yells came from all of them before the party was over. At the end of the night, I sold hundreds of dollars of toys. It was the most successful and exciting night I had ever had.

My next party I decided to invite couples. Once they arrived, they all stripped down to nothing but a smile. Each couple picked a toy or two or three that they wanted to try out before buying. Some had cock rings and others had edible panties, but they wanted me to get the party started.

I took off my bikini and got into my sex swing. I was laying back slightly in it with my legs spread wide.

I told Jake that he could use any of the toys on me that would excite him. He picked a vibrator with a rotating head. "How about this one? I bet I can make you cum with this baby."

"Try to only drive me crazy, not make me come," I said. "Give more people a chance." His partner came over to me, pinched my nipples and put on nipple clamps. I didn't think I would like them, but they were exciting. Jake turned on the vibrator, and at first moved it over my clit and in my hole for a moment than back over my clit. "Put it in me."

Jake did just that letting the vibrations and rotation drive me to almost orgasm, then stopped and pulled it out of me. I was sad until I saw what was next for me. The other couples watched contently, all the men were very erect with excitement.

John took some edible lotion that gets warm on contact, and put it on my clit. He kneeled between my legs and rubbed it around at first, the warmth really excited me. Then he used his tongue and licked my pussy and teased my clit. I wanted to come so bad I ached, but just as I started to shake, he stopped.

All of a sudden everyone got toys off the table that they wanted to try, it was the same feeding frenzy that I saw at the other party.

I looked at the ten people at this party who were now pleasuring each other with toys. Some couples were in their own world, and some watched others.

Judy, John's partner, came over to me with a little machine called the Magic Tongue, and John grabbed one of the bigger dildos. John smiled as he shoved the dildo into my pussy. In and out it went into me while the swing moved to help the thrusts. Then Judy held the swing so she could put the Magic Tongue on my clit. Within a few seconds I screamed in orgasm, Judy and John left me to please each other.

Again the party sold a lot of toys, and everyone went home very satisfied. Friday came and I threw another party. This time I wanted to teach the men of the couples to please their women in a different way. It was vibrator and ice night—I had buckets of ice out and the website's new smooth plastic vibrators that were about seven inches long and two and a half inches wide. They not only vibrated, they got cold with ice cubes that you put inside them. Plus the movement of the ice going up and down as the vibrator was thrusting in and out was even more of a turn on.

"Can I have a volunteer?" I asked, and David spoke up first.

"Take Janelle. I want to watch you turn her on," he said. His cock was already hard.

Janelle walked over to me and sat in the convenient swing. David helped spread her legs for me and for everyone to watch. First, I took a piece of ice and moved it over her abs, then up over her firm large breasts and around her hard nipples. Then I moved the ice down between her legs and slipped it into her pussy. She jumped a little, but then said, "Wow, that's great."

"David, lick her pussy," I said. I must admit it really did turn me on to see how excited I was able to make people. Their pleasure became my pleasure.

He dove between her legs licking and sucking all of the melting ice from her, as she moaned in pleasure.

I put two pieces of ice into the chilled vibrator, and moved David out of the way. He was content watching. I turned the cold vibrator on and slowly thrust it deep into her pussy. She was so wet that I could hear her sounds of pleasure, David pushed the swing, so each time it helped the vibrator moved harder and faster into her.

"Make me come!" She yelled. I knew her clit was twice as hard with the ice in her. I slipped the vibrator out, held it to her clit and she screamed immediately in orgasm. David moved between her legs and stuck his hard cock in her. She shook in what looked like a continual orgasm until he thrust really hard and came in her.

At that point the rest of the couples started to use the ice on their partners teasing them before using the cold vibrators in their pussies to make them cum. As I watched the toy party, I took a vibrator and sat on the couch to satisfy myself. I was so horny at that point that I ached to come. One after another, the women came before their men screwed them to another orgasm.

Needless to say all of my cold vibrators sold that night. I had finally found my niche in the marketing world, not to mention some exciting times and great toys. No one was ever dissatisfied at my toy parties, including me.

My Adventures

Can you come up with other exciting ways to use your vibrator?

....
....
....
....
....
....
....
....
....
....
....
....
....
....
....
....
....
....
....